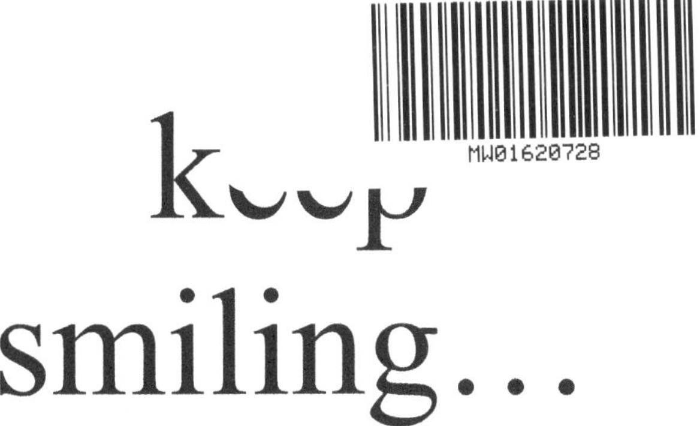

keep smiling…

What to do when your world turns upside down

By Sandy Sheaffer

Published by: Dewey Productions
2701 SW 139
Oklahoma City, OK 73170
405-692-8811
www.DeweyProductions.com
or email: sheaffersandy@cox.net

ISBN #978-0-9823364-2-7

Dedicated to:

Anyone who has

ever been Hurt

Table of Contents

Chapter ____________ Page

Introduction

When I first started thinking about writing this book, I jotted down several ideas. As I wrote, I thought of more. I also realized that this was a book I was *supposed* to write. It was almost as if the Lord was telling me that this book is the reason I went through everything I've been through. I love that! I have always prayed for God to make my mess my message, and here you go – my message in book form.

This book is written somewhat like the Bible. Keep in mind I use God, Jesus, and sometimes the Holy Spirit, interchangeably. I was taught they are the Holy Trinity. It's like talking about the egg. The shell, the yolk, and the white all make up the egg, whether you are talking about them separately or together.

This book is made from journal entries, letters, bits of wisdom handed down from my parents, parts of Sunday School lessons, and mainly life lessons learned along the way – really never meant for others to see. Somehow now, I want to share. I want to hopefully help someone else along life's way. Let's face it, life can get messy. Wait, life *IS* messy!

So, here is my messy life - at least the painful parts, yet with a wonderful, gigantic concoction of how in painful moments, Jesus is very near, and life is magnificent. One of my favorite mottos is:

Life is like pizza.
Even when it's bad, it's good!

It's true. It can even be horrible and wonderful all at the same time. As I have traveled life's road, I have learned to keep smiling. I have learned to "wash my face," as Rachel Hollis puts it. I have put my big girl (and yes, sometimes bigger than I care to admit) panties on and have learned to keep smiling.

When I say to keep smiling, I mean that we know the ending of the book. We know that Christ turns all things for good. We know that we win. We know that even in the difficult trials of life that Jesus will be with us. We know that even in our desperation we can find a deeper relationship than we ever dreamed possible if we keep going and don't stop. Yes, sometimes we have to plaster that smile on and just take another step. It doesn't mean we are being fake. We are just believing that even though we can't see the end result at the moment, we know that everything will work out for our good. I also don't want you to think that having negative emotions is a bad thing. Life can be tough and we all have to learn how to navigate through those difficult times.

As always with my books, I am compelled to share this. I believe God is driving it. My prayer is that someone will be in the middle of the worst situation in their life, not knowing what to do or where to turn, and this will encourage them to turn to Jesus, trust the end result to Him, and to keep smiling. It is always helpful to know, like the 3 Hebrew boys, that someone made it through the pain and has come out on the other side without even the smell of smoke!

We need to hear that there was a fourth man in the fire. Jesus was in the furnace right beside them. They were going through the absolute worst experience of their lives, yet in the flames, Jesus was alongside. That is comforting! However, he didn't put out the fire. Those are the stories we love to read and hear about again and again. We can take bad situations if we know that Jesus walks with us and sees us through to the victorious end!

This book is also a book of hope. Hope is expectation that Jesus will be with you during your crisis. Hope that He will comfort you through the darkest valley. Hope that He will help you make it through the night and hang on until the morning… and in that morning - just as the Bible tells us, there will be joy!

Perhaps this book will help to heal another's broken heart. Perhaps someone will read it and it will help them to understand what to do in the middle of their darkness... And in my wildest dreams, perhaps those who read it, will be able to do what I did and…

keep smiling!

God bless you and keep you,
God smile on you and gift you,
God look you full in the face
and make you prosper.
Numbers 6:24-26 MSG

Chapter One –
My First Venture into Darkness

In looking back, I see now what God was doing. I no longer see the pain. I see my heartache taking me to a deeper place where God could actually use me and perfect my gifts. I am able to see with 20/20 vision. God sees things this way *all* of the time. My tiny perspective of the world isn't able to do that. I only see my pain, my sadness, and my life not turning out as *I* want it to.

My perfect little childhood was wonderful until my happiness turned to sadness. Celia and I had been best friends since I was 5. Now she was moving away. Who would I play with? What would I do with my time? I was so sad. I was also bored. My best friend had left with her family for Africa.

I was only 8 years old. In that day and time, there was no internet or facetime and no way to correspond with my friend, except through letters which took approximately two weeks or longer to get to her. Then I had to wait the two weeks for her answer to get back to me. It seemed to my 8 year old mind that a continent away, was actually a life time away. She was gone.

Our neighborhood had always been so full of fun! There were seven of us who would hang out and play. My older sister, Vicki, and I were rarely in the house. Vicki mainly played with Sherry and Kathy, who were both her age. My best friend was Celia, who was one year younger than I was. Celia had two older sisters, Mary Zoe and Beverly. Mary Zoe was a year older than my sister, Vicki, and Beverly was one year older than me. Norma lived one street over but was usually with the rest of us.

What a fun group! We played tag, hide and seek, listened to Beatles music, and found fun wherever we were. Once we put on a show for the neighborhood with real curtains. "The Beatles" performed in that show! My dad made us wooden guitars that he had jig sawed to look like each of John, Paul, and George's guitars. He then used pop bottle tops painted and attached for the guitar knobs. Another dad made us curtains on a pulley. They were made of bed sheets and hung on a rope. Believe it or not, they could open and close. It was quite a performance! Some sang and some danced. Oh how I wish we had iPhone video back then.

Once the seven of us rode the train alone down to Fort Worth. We took the Six Flags Inn van from the train station to the hotel. We spent the night without our parents, went to Six Flags the next day, then rode the train home. We had an absolute blast. I know, I know - What were all of our parents thinking? I'm sure they would just tell you that it was a different day and time – and it was!

When Celia and her family moved away, almost half of our neighborhood group, 3 or the 7, were gone. It wasn't the same. In my boredom I began playing the piano. Practicing on the piano is how I dealt with my best friend moving to Africa.

I look back and see that God used my sorrow and my loneliness, and led me to the piano. It was during those first months and years that I played the piano and sang, and without even realizing it, I practiced.

> *It's funny how the grief and isolation*
> *of what I was going through*
> *became a conduit for one of*
> *my life's greatest talents.*

My mother was worried about me because I practiced so much. In less than three years, I caught up with my piano teacher! She had given me all she knew. That makes me giggle now. I loved her as a teacher, but I had gotten to where I didn't want to play what she wanted me to. I wanted to play new music.

Finally, in the seventh grade, my mom made me a bargain. If I tried out for the choir pianist and got it, she would allow me to quit taking lessons. She would spend the same amount on new music that she was spending on my lessons. I could teach myself. So I did it! I became the choir pianist, and thus at 12 years old began my illustrious career of piano playing for various choirs and groups.

In my opinion I believe that's one of the reasons I am a good sight reader! I couldn't wait to go pick out new music to learn! I would say, it is difficult to be a kid and deal with depression. I was lonely, downhearted, and couldn't see *any* good coming from this season of my life. Don't get me wrong, when I was at school, I had many friends there, but when I came home, there was no one to play with and no reason to go outside.

Luckily, a new friend, Diane Craig, moved in a few months later, and we became fast friends. In fact we are still friends today! In a funny turn of events, she even worked at a company with me in my later years. God is so good to allow people to come and go at just the right times! So even though it was a difficult path, it led me in the most beautiful direction. Playing the piano is something I absolutely adore doing!

I played for my junior high choir in 7th, 8th and 9th grades! In high school, I again became the glee club choir pianist. I played for the Glee Club in 10th and 11th grade. My senior year, the choir director forced me to choose between taking my leadership class for being the head cheerleader and being the pianist. I chose leadership, and sadly had to give up my place at the piano. It wasn't a tough decision for me.

> *However, although I didn't know it at the time, my piano playing days for choir were far from over!*

In high school my sweetheart, Mike Sheaffer, who later became my husband, invited me to go to church with him. His parents were ministers at a local Assembly of God church, so he had to be at church twice on Sunday and on Wednesday evenings. If I wanted to be with him, I had to go to church.

Mike's mom called my mom a few months into our relationship and told her exactly that!!! I still have the notes from their conversation. My wise mother did not agree to the terms. She said she would leave that up to me. She also told Bonnie that we always went as a family to our church, so I couldn't attend on Sunday mornings. That's exactly what I did.

I did not attend even one Sunday morning service until the Sunday one week after our wedding! Anyway, about a year later, I was sitting in the choir room because my husband played the drums for the Sunday morning choir. Their piano player did not show up. Homer Bair, the choir director, figured she would be there by the time the choir performed. She didn't show up, which was highly unusual. Homer was talking to Pastor Sheaffer about cancelling the choir song. I could see how concerned he was. I walked over and whispered to him that I could play it.

The shocked look on his face told me he didn't really *believe* that I could play it. He wanted to believe me. He said, "We don't have time to rehearse it or anything!" I told him I knew that, but I had been sitting there throughout the rehearsal and knew without a doubt, I could play it. He was trepidatious, but agreed. I was nervous and prayed quickly under my breath for God to help me to do my best. Homer began counting to begin the song… He was unaware of the many years of practice with school choirs that had preceded this moment.

I didn't miss one note! I didn't miss a beat! Homer was ecstatic and so was I! To say I was smiling would be an understatement! I was proud of myself and so was my husband. Homer came over and congratulated me, and quickly asked if I would be his backup piano player! Before that time, he had no idea I could even play.

It's funny how the Lord makes room for our talents at the perfect time and place. If you are practicing and preparing for an opportunity, God will provide it. You may not be able to see it coming. Be hopeful. Don't look at the circumstance, especially if there is pain and sadness. Try to look at it with the 20/20 vision of the Lord. Recognize that He is doing something that will matter later, possibly much later. It can be hard. Humans are self-centered and want what they want right then and there. We don't like waiting for things. God, on the other hand, is extremely patient.

Proverbs 18:16 NKJV says, A man's gift makes room for him… Dr. Miles Munroe explains it by saying:

God has put a gift or talent in every person the world will make room for. It is this gift that will enable you to fulfill your vision. It will make a way for you in life. It is in exercising this gift that you will find real fulfillment, purpose, and contentment in your work. It is interesting to note that the Bible does not say that man's education makes room for him, but that his gift does.

Years later in 1982, I became the choir piano player. I was ready because God had prepared me. All those hours during a lonely time in my childhood finally bore some fruit. There was no way I could have known that the Lord would take the hours of practice in my sadness and turn it into a true ministry for His kingdom. It would have been so much easier to get through. It would have made sense, but you see that is not how God works.

He takes those difficult times in the valley and later makes it all make sense.

So in looking back, I no longer see the pain. I see the results. If you are in a time of depression and darkness, lift up your head. Do not despair.

God knows exactly where you are.

If you are the best singer in the choir, yet you're not getting any solos – just hang on. If you are stuck in a dead-end job and feel like no one notices how hard you work, keep up the good work. If you are in the depths of depression and worry whether you will make it out alive, hold on. If you feel like you are supposed to be leading, yet you are in prison, like Joseph – stick it out.

Your time will come. Perhaps Jesus is giving you time to hone your skills and talents for something bigger and better in the future that He can use for His kingdom.

Learn to be patient. So work hard, look for God's presence in the darkness, and don't forget to…

keep smiling…

**Old people are distinguished
by grandchildren;
children take pride in their parents.
Proverbs 17:6 MSG**

Chapter Two –
Don't Drink and Drive

I lost my grandfather in 1982. He was my dad's father, the one who taught me to play piano and sing. He would put one of us in his lap and play the organ for us when we visited after church on Sundays. Neither of my sisters sat there as often or as long as I did. I would say, "Play it again, Grandad!" and he would. He played *She'll Be Coming 'Round the Mountain* too many times to even mention. Sometimes Terri, Vicki and I would dance around the room. Sometimes we would sing. Sometimes he played Christmas Carols or Hymns. Sometimes we would play albums. I distinctly remember, *Won't You Come Home Bill Bailey?* There was always music playing.

I found out years later that Grandad, John H. Spaan Jr., had been an organist for silent movies when he was a young man. He was an excellent organist, and frankly I could have sat there all day watching him play. The amount of time and energy he spent with me, was not wasted. He did it because he loved me, and he enjoyed watching my sisters and cousins be amused with his talent. Grandad never really knew the huge impact he had on my life. He knew I played for the church and I'm sure he loved that, but he died before I could fully express my gratitude.

He was killed by a drunk driver in 1982, who broadsided his huge Cadillac, when Grandad pulled out from the bank. It was the middle of the day. Too early for most people to even start drinking, but this guy had several (7 if I remember correctly) DUI's. Grandad was his latest transgression in a long list of alcohol related accidents. I was devastated.

These were generally such happy days. I had just found out I was pregnant again with child number two. We already had a son who was 2 ½ years old. We called him Doc. His name is actually Michael Dan so his initials are M.D., as in a medical doctor, thus the nickname. Exciting things were happening at church, too.

Our church had been invited to come to Malawi, Africa. Life President Banda had heard one of Pastor Sheaffer's tapes sent there through our tape ministry, headed by Jim and Shirley Outon. They would tape every service. They would choose one, and send cassette tapes to our Assembly of God missionaries once a month. Because of this, we had a group of singers and players headed over there to build a church.

I was supposed to go, but due to the pregnancy, we decided it was too risky. We had never been there before and really had no idea what it would be like. I would also have to take several vaccinations which might put the baby in jeopardy. The trip was two weeks after the loss of Grandad.

The loss of Grandad left a void in me. He was 80, so he had lived a good life, however, it was too soon as far as I was concerned. I think the reason it devastated me so much was because I had never lost anyone in my inner circle. My husband had lost a couple of grandparents, but it wasn't the same as losing mine. We had moved into a condo because the house we had purchased was being renovated and wasn't ready yet.

Lying in bed, alone, every night for two weeks while Mike was in Africa, I had a lot of time to think and to pray. I kept trying to make sense of it all. Sometimes that is impossible. This time I decided this was simply an opportunity to draw closer to God, and that's what I did. I started attending the Women's Ministry and reading my Bible more.

One night, as I lay in bed after a night of preaching from R. W. Shambach, I prayed for the baptism in the Holy Spirit. It was a scary thing to me. Being raised as an Episcopalian, I didn't really understand speaking in tongues. After all, we were God's "frozen chosen!" We didn't play loud music or speak in tongues or raise our hands to praise the Lord. I had gotten comfortable with raising my hands, or maybe just one hand, to praise the Lord! I loved the loud exciting music!

But the tongues…

That was scary.

That was unknown.

Why was that even necessary?

Somehow in my sorrow,
it didn't matter what or why.
I just wanted whatever
God had to give me.

I prayed and received the Baptism of the Holy Spirit that night, and began to speak in a heavenly prayer language. It was incredible! I realize some people don't believe in this. I do. I was raised in the Episcopal Church so this was *the* most difficult difference for me of being in an Assembly of God church. Everything else seemed to align quite nicely. I just wasn't sure about this Holy Spirit thing. I certainly wasn't ready to speak in tongues.

By this point I thought it was fine if others wanted that gift, but I didn't think I needed it. Grandad's death, and walking through that valley, taught me otherwise. I needed direction and help through it.

If you are not the religious type, feel free to go ahead and skip to chapter 3, page 28. For those that want to read my entire story, continue reading how I received the baptism of the Holy Spirit and prayed in tongues for the first time.

It was during the difficult time and of losing my beloved grandfather. I needed help. I needed more. I prayed for God to help me. I prayed for Jesus to comfort me, but that scripture in John 16:7 where Jesus calls the Holy Spirit our comforter, made me feel that I *did* need the Holy Spirit. At this point *I* needed *Him*. I feel some explanation is needed here for those who may not have studied this before.

In John 14:16-17 scripture says,

> *And I will pray the Father, and He will give you another Helper, that He may abide with you forever – the Spirit of truth, whom the world cannot receive, because it neither sees Him nor knows Him; but you know Him, for He dwells with you and will be in you.*

Two words are important here: another and helper. I like the way the article I'm using here, "*The Holy Spirit our Helper: Parakletos*," explains it:

a) 'allos' – which speaks of 'another one but of the same sort / kind'

b) 'heteros' – which speaks of 'another of a different sort / kind'

If I have a chair and I change it for 'another' chair, I can either get one exactly the same – and although it is still 'another chair', it is another one of the same kind; or I can get 'another chair' that is completely different.

It is still another chair but it is another one of a different kind.

In the English we use the same word 'another' in both instances, but in the Greek there were two words to show this delicate difference.

The first of these, allos, is the one that is used in John 14:16 in reference to the Holy Spirit.

Jesus is saying that the Holy Spirit is another of the exact same kind as me: He'll be to you what I have been to you! Jesus was saying that The Holy Spirit will be in your life, everything *He* was to the disciples while on this earth, however it will be better for you because He will be in you and with you at all times.

We do not lose out by Jesus' physical departure, rather we gain with the presence of the Holy Spirit with and in us now.

So since Jesus spoke of 'another' that would be the same kind, I believe this means he is sending a person. Someone we can have a relationship with. But as with any type of relationship, we can choose to have one or not.

The second 'another' tells us of a different kind. This is the Holy Spirit as a helper. Do you need help? Are there times you feel alone? Perhaps you have even felt God wasn't near.

It is in those times that we need a helper. Someone to guide us and speak to us throughout this journey called life. We again get to choose.

Do you want to be out there all alone?

Would you prefer to have a helper you can call on when times get rough?

Having been through some really rough times, I can tell you from experience that having the Holy Spirit to call on and ask for His help is essential for anyone who is a disciple of Christ.

Do you need help?
Are there times you feel alone?
Perhaps you have even felt God wasn't near.
It is in those times that we need a helper.
Someone to guide us and speak
to us throughout this journey called life.

Let's face it, the world can be cruel and harsh. We can feel alone. We can feel afraid. We can be left to wonder if life has dealt us a blow that we cannot handle. I believe the Holy Spirit is for those times that Jesus told us in John 14, He wouldn't leave us alone. In John 15:26 NIV, Jesus called the Holy Spirit our Advocate and it is capitalized. "When the Advocate comes, whom I will send to you from the Father…" This word, Advocate, means,

> *one who pleads the cause of another; one who defends or maintains a cause…; one who supports or promotes the interests of a cause or group.*

In the NKJV for the same scripture, it is translated helper and it is capitalized as if a proper name, "But when the *Helper* comes, whom I shall send to you from the Father,..." Later, Jesus calls him the Comforter.

Nevertheless I tell you the truth; It is expedient for you that I go away; for if I go not away, the Comforter will not come unto you; but if I depart, I will send him unto you. John 16:7 KJV

Jesus knew that it was more beneficial for us if He physically left, so that the Holy Spirit could come. Read this powerful translation for the Holy Spirit:

> *However, I am telling you nothing but the truth when I say it is profitable (good, expedient, advantageous) for you that I go away. Because if I do not go away, the Comforter (Counselor, Helper, Advocate, Intercessor, Strengthener, Standby) will not come to you [into close fellowship with you]; but if I go away, I will send Him to you [to be in close fellowship with you].*
> *John 16:7 AMPC*

The Holy Spirit is for us. Jesus sent Him to help us! Some synonyms for help are: assist, benefit, aid, support, comfort, etc.

Who wouldn't benefit from a great counselor?

Who, at times, doesn't need a helper?

Who wouldn't want an advocate if you were heading into a courtroom where someone was accusing you of something?

We all could benefit from a strengthener, an intercessor, and a standby. As with most gifts provided by

God, our free will becomes involved. We decide what we want to invite into our lives. God is the quintessential gentlemen. He never forces Himself on us. He allows us to choose.

My advice is simple. Invite the Holy Spirit in. Open yourself up to whatever God has for you. You may not know what the future holds, but a helper along this unknown road is really advantageous. Try it! Pray this simple prayer out loud and to God:

Lord, please hear my prayer.

Jesus, I believe You are the Son of God. I know you came to earth, lived a sinless life, were crucified and buried for three days before rising from the dead and ascending into Heaven to sit at the right hand of God. Forgive me of my sins. I ask that you send the Holy Spirit to me. Help me to understand that He is the third person in the blessed Trinity. I am asking for the Holy Spirit to overtake and live in me so that I may be a true follower of Jesus Christ. I ask for the gifts of the Spirit to live in me and allow those around me to see them at work in my life. Lord, we ask it all in your name.

Amen.

After you pray this prayer, just close this book for a few minutes and pray.

Wait on the Lord.

Don't forget that He takes His time.

He's not instant.

We live in an "instant" society, wanting everything to happen quickly. The Holy Spirit comes at His own pace. His timing is perfect timing. You may have to ask several times, for several days, weeks, months, or so on. You may need to pray this prayer every day for a period of time.

Pray again.

Ask again.

Keep asking.

If you are struggling, remember the scripture in Matthew 5: 24 that says:

> *If you enter your place of worship and, about to make an offering, you suddenly remember a grudge a friend has against you, abandon your offering, leave immediately, go to this friend and make things right. Then and only then, come back and work things out with God.*
> *Matt. 5: 24 MSG*

It is always good to make sure you have done everything to clear the way for Him. Everyone's experience is different. Just know that Jesus wants you to have the Holy Spirit. He said so in John 14:26 MSG,

> *The Friend, the Holy Spirit whom the Father will send at my request, will make everything plain to you. He will remind you of all the things I have told you. I'm leaving you well and whole. That's my parting gift to you. Peace. I don't leave you the way you're used to being left—feeling abandoned, bereft. So don't be upset. Don't be distraught. John 14:26 MSG*

Another translation says,

> *But the Helper, the Holy Spirit, whom the Father will send in My name, He will teach you all things, and bring to your remembrance all things that I said to you. John 14:26 NKJV*

I'll be praying for this book to be a blessing and hopefully be the touchpoint for many who have never invited Him in, to do so. In Jesus' name.

I believe the Holy Spirit can guide you and speak to you in supernatural ways. There are often times in my life I don't know what to pray, or how to pray for something. That's when I speak in tongues.

> *This divine connection with God, allows my heart to speak to Him when words escape me.*

I don't believe that not having the Holy Spirit or not speaking in tongues will keep you out of heaven, but it just makes the journey here a bit easier! So my question is: Why wouldn't you want it?

I love how Jesus can meet you in the valley of the shadow of death. Scripture say He gives life. Trust me, when you are walking that road, you need life in the valley of death.

> *He can show up in the darkest moments of your life and bring light to your life that you never expected.*

ASK and He can give you an extraordinary gift!

He can bless you in ways that bring you peace in the midst of the storm. When you ask, He can give you the ability in the darkest of times to…

keep smiling…

Pay close attention, friend,
to what your father tells you;
never forget what you learned
at your mother's knee.
Wear their counsel like flowers in your hair,
like rings on your fingers.
Proverbs 1:8-9 MSG

Chapter Three – Who's Your Daddy?

In September 1984 I lost my grandmother. We called her Nanny, and she was my dad's mother. Looking back, I realize that I'm very much like her. When she was living, I generally stayed away from her, but not because I didn't like her. I think it was because she was always with my older sister, Vicki, and then when Terri, the baby, came along, she spent a lot of time with her too. Since no one was around Grandad, I would gravitate to him. However, I was continually watching Nanny.

Nanny was always laughing. She was always there at our recitals and games. She never missed a trip to the lake. This woman taught me the meaning of fun. She could take a normal event and turn it into a party. She loved hosting parties and family gatherings. This is interesting because even though I wasn't "with" her, she taught me how to enjoy life, host parties, make people feel welcome, and how to love and enjoy family. Don't ever think that because you consider someone doesn't like you or want to be with you that you aren't making an impact. God can use those times to make a huge impact on a life – on a spectator.

Think about that! I wasn't in her lap. I didn't sleep in bed with her whenever my sisters and I spent the night. Yet her impact upon me was enormous. Watching her from afar, perhaps I learned more from her than even my two sisters, who were always in her lap. I believe it when I read things like,

> *"Fathers, be careful what you say to your children, but be more careful what you do." Author Unknown.*

Children often watch what you do far more than listening to what you say! Children are more likely to do what you do than do what you say.

When I think back about Nanny, I smile. I can't help it! I hear her laughing. I see her eyes sparkling. Even when she lost Grandad, she made the best of it. She traveled with her widowed and single friends. She played bridge. She worked at the church. She helped with Thanksgiving and Christmas dinners. For most of my life, she had hosted those events. We always went to Nanny's house. It was never a question of where it was going to be. We knew it would be at Nanny's. She loved it! She loved her place being the center of our family. She was the gravitational pull for all of us!

As my kids grew older, I realized I was like that too. I wanted my kids to be at my house. I loved that we had the swimming pool. Have you ever noticed that if kids have water, they're happy? Well, me too! I think maybe I got this love for life from Nanny. In the previous few years before her death, her health had been declining. My mother had told me stories of her not remembering that Grandad was gone. She would sometimes talk to him or claim that he was in the room. My dad would want to "bring her back to reality." Mother, however, would let her go on about it. Mom even thought, perhaps it was true – that Grandad *was* in the room. I know I believe in the supernatural. It could have been possible that Grandad was there.

One night she was especially bad. Mom told me she had come for dinner with them. She kept saying things that didn't make sense. Finally, my dad couldn't take it anymore. He told her that she was obviously tired and he needed to take her home. Dad drove her to her apartment and tucked her in bed. Nanny had had a few mini-strokes and Dad was afraid she was having another.

Isn't it interesting that as our elderly parent's age, the roles reverse? The child becomes the caregiver. Here was my dad tucking his mom into bed as if she's a 3 year old, and I guess in some ways, she was. Dad was very worried about her. He did not like her traveling between reality and fantasyland. Because he was worried, he went the next morning to check on her. She had passed away in the night.

We were all so sad, however, we found peace that she was with Grandad, her parents, her sister, and other friends who had gone before. We also reconsidered whether she had been in fantasyland the night before. Maybe Grandad *had* come to get her.

Soon after her death, one of my sisters had a dream that Nanny came to see her to say goodbye. When she woke up from their conversation, she was sitting up on the bed with Kleenexes all around her from when she was crying while they talked. Was it real? I believe so. I believe God gives us what we need. Something similar happened to me when my ex-mother-in-law passed away years later in 2011. Obviously my sister needed to say goodbye. We were all grieving the loss of our precious mom and grandmother. One week later on the following Tuesday morning, my dad's brother, Gary, finally got on a plane to head back home.

That same day which was one week to the day after Nanny died, on Tuesday, September 18, 1984, I was in my husband's office at Crossroads Cathedral, now known as Crossroads Church OKC. Someone called and told Mike dad passed out in his garage and was headed to the hospital. This certainly was unusual and quite scary. Lucky for me, Doc was at preschool so I grabbed Duke, who was 1 ½ years old, and we headed to Saint Anthony Hospital. I knew that's where he would be headed because Dad's best friend, Dr. Honick, was a cardiologist there.

He had given Dad a complete heart health checkup less than two weeks prior and Dad had passed with flying colors, so I knew it wasn't a heart attack. However, when I ran into the emergency room at Saint Anthony's, they had no record of my Dad being there. Now I was worried. I knew that an ambulance would take you to the hospital of your choice *if* you were doing okay, however, if it was life threatening, they would take you to the nearest hospital.

I jumped back in the car with my baby, and drove to Baptist Hospital, now known as Integris. I hurried to the E.R. and was immediately directed to a beautiful room off and away from the actual waiting room. How nice, I thought. I didn't realize Baptist Hospital had such a lovely waiting area. Mom was there and she looked worried. I was too. No one had been in to tell us anything. Soon Vicki arrived and some others. To be honest it is a blur.

As the minutes passed, I looked around and realized this was all bad. The waiting, the beautiful room, the fact that no one had been in to talk to us, were not good signs. Somehow, I knew Dad was gone. Finally, T arrived and she quickly strode over to Mom, telling her that everything was going to be okay and that Dad would be fine. I was behind Mom shaking my head no. I didn't want Terri to give Mom any false hope. I think they were waiting for my little sister to arrive, because shortly after everyone was there, someone came in and told us that he was gone.

Wait. What?!? What do you mean - gone? My Dad was only 56 years old. He had been given a clean bill of health not two weeks earlier! How was this possible? We sat there in shock and in silence. The nurse asked if we wanted to see him. Vicki, my sister who is the nurse, said yes. We lined up shortly after she explained that we could only be in there for a few seconds to say our goodbyes.

We walked in. I saw my Dad laying there with a breathing apparatus in his mouth that a nurse was hand pumping oxygen into him. I saw his beautiful crystal blue eyes. They were partially open, as if he were just falling asleep. I reached out to touch him and realized he wasn't there at all. His spirit had already gone. I'm not sure any of us were crying yet. I don't think it had sunken in. Somewhere in all the hubbub, my husband Mike, had arrived too. We all went back to the beautiful waiting room and just stared at one another. Mom wanted to go home. There was nothing else we could do here, so we went to Mom's house. There we cried. We tried to imagine a world without John Spaan in it. We couldn't.

Grief is strange. You can be crying one minute and then laughing the next. We had just buried Nanny the previous week. Dad had been working on going through her things. Later we wondered if the electronic engraver that he used to etch her name on the bottom of her silver trinkets caused him to have a heart attack. What did it matter? He was gone forever.

It was strange though. I kept thinking he would walk in from the garage with his big personality and fun loving baritone, and be looking for his mug that said "Dad," that was always sitting on the refrigerator shelf where the water comes out, explaining what car he was currently working on, but he never did. It was now only about 10:30 AM. Time had slowed to a crawl. Duke was a wonderful distraction. We would do things for him then cry for a bit.

Through all of this Mom was so strong. She really didn't cry. It was surreal. We had just been through a terrible loss, one week to the day with Nanny, but we never expected this. Several weeks later we learned that he actually *did* have a heart attack. He had an arrhythmia and his heart just stopped with no explanation. His dear friend, Dr. Honick, even watched the whole autopsy to see for himself what he had missed. Dad had told us he didn't want a funeral, so it became important to do what he wanted. The four of us - Mom, Vicki, T and I - did go to All Soul's Episcopal Church for their Wednesday morning service because they called Dad by name and prayed for him and for us. That was as close as we came to a funeral.

Several months down the road, we all four, expressed remorse that we didn't have a service to celebrate his life and have a certain point of reference to grieve together. Up until then I had always thought funerals were for the dead, but I discovered the hard way that these services are actually for those who are left behind. I also found out that the living should make the decisions – even if those decisions are different than the person who died. The deceased person is already gone and doesn't need anything.

I remember that evening going over to Dan and Bonnie's with Mike and the boys. Dan came over and hugged me so tight. I began to cry. He said, "I'll be your Dad." It was extremely comforting to me. Up until I lost my dad, I thought my dad hung the moon. He was always there whenever I needed him, with words of wisdom and help in any way I needed it; whether it was to fix a broken down car or just moral support. It was through this loss I truly found that God is my father.

*...You **are** my Father, My God, and the rock of my salvation. Psalm 89:26*

The Bible says this, but do we really believe it? I had to begin living it.

During this time, there was so much going on in my own life. Earlier that year in February, Mike and I had gone into business with his sister, Terri, and her husband, Glen Smith, in a Mexican restaurant named Mario's. It was located in Oklahoma City on South Shields and 92nd Street. We had joined, based on projections provided to us by Glen. Looking back, this was the first of many mistakes! We didn't want to miss out on all the money they would be making. One problem was their marriage. Mike had a serious talk with Terri before we linked up with them in this venture. We wanted to be sure that she would be staying with him. They had always had a fairly unstable and volatile relationship. We knew if the marriage wasn't going to last, then the partnership would be in jeopardy. The previous year Terri and Glen had a second son, and the family hoped this would solidify the marriage. Terri assured Mike that she would be staying with Glen for "the long haul."

Well, long story short, the marriage didn't last. They split up in May of this same year, and Glen was so angry that he immediately began taking money out of the cash register. He even purchased a new Porsche and a Rolex watch! During the separation he stole Terri's Cadillac out of the parking garage while she was at work. She called the police and they later found it. She knew it had been Glen who took it. On another night trying to get to the children, he got so mad that he rammed his truck through Terri's garage door. Terri called the police and then she called Mike. Mike and our dear friend, Dan Garland, rushed to the scene, taking our gun with them! I remember being so scared! I thought perhaps Glen might kill all of them! Thankfully, it was resolved peacefully. God is good.

Shortly after the garage door incident, Terri got the temporary order for the dissolution of their marriage. Because of the temporary order of their divorce, with the three of us - Terri, Mike and I, we had 75% control of the restaurant. Glen was furious! We had control of *his* restaurant, and frankly the three of us weren't restaurateurs. After a few months of trying to run it, while busy with our other lives and then having the pipes burst during a freeze, it was only a matter of months until we closed the doors for good on December 31, 1984.

This is all pretty heavy, so let me throw in a good dad joke:

> Why do chicken coops only have 2 doors? Because if they had 4, they would be called chicken sedans!!!

Dads are awesome. They give you a hero to look up to when you're young. They give you someone to run to when mom just won't listen! They give you someone to be embarrassed about when they wear white socks with sandals! They give you someone to call when your car breaks down in the pouring rain! That is, if they are good dads. If they aren't, they can inflict life-long wounds. Their void in a child's life cannot be filled by anyone else. This goes for moms too!

Father's Day is especially brutal. I miss my dad every day, but his memory is front and center when I see all the Father's Day advertisements. Every daughter I have spoken to, mourns the loss of her Daddy. It is a tough time to go through. If you are in that season, my prayer is that you will find solace in knowing you still have your heavenly Father. Invite Him to be your dad.

If you still have your dad here, call him or go see him, or better yet, have him for dinner or plan a trip to get together. What I wouldn't do for just one more conversation with my dad. Losing my Dad and Nanny seven days apart was almost too much! I felt surrounded by death and sadness. Sorrow was my new friend. There was a pressure on my chest and a broken heart inside of it. I felt as if I had been left for dead in the valley of death.

Those dark days sent me to my Bible. Isn't that what we are supposed to do? Read the Bible. I read and reread the scriptures about Jesus who was left for dead after Calvary. I am sure the disciples felt like I did… but the story wasn't over. They just needed to hold on. I had to hold on too. I had to find my purpose for living and start living it. While I was doing that, I just needed to read the Bible, talk to my heavenly Father, and…

keep smiling…

And he said unto them,
Go ye into all the world,
and preach the gospel
to every creature.
Mark 16:15 KJV

Chapter 4 –
Africa is Calling

In 1985 I went on my first mission trip to Africa. I had been to Cartagena, Columbia, and 2 different places in Jamaica on mission trips, but I had never traveled this far. Jesus told us to preach the gospel and we know that the gospel is the Good News! So we are to go into the world and speak about the Good News. Basically this Good News is that Jesus is our Savior – He is the Christ. We are also to share the glory that is to come and tell about His second coming. Most of us need to know that it doesn't matter what your history is, what you've done, what sins you may have committed, how dark your heart is, - the Good News is that He loves you anyway. Jesus gave a clear command in Matt 28:19-20:

> *GO therefore and make disciples of all the nations, baptizing them in the name of the Father and of the Son and of the Holy Spirit, teaching them to observe all things I have commanded you; I am with you always, even to the end of the age. Matt. 28:19-20*

When that happens, they too are charged with the great commission, so it is a circle of life. We are to GO! So that is exactly what I decided to do. I was apprehensive and there were many decisions to make and things to do. Who would keep my children? Where should we have a will drawn up? What if something happens to both of us and my children were left with no parents? The mind can come up with all sorts of reasons not to GO, but I was commanded. Command means instructed. I was basically told by Jesus to GO. God would take care of us and our children! Mike had always returned to us and so would I!

Up until now, I had stayed at home with my babies. As you have already read, I was pregnant, so I wasn't able to go. Duke, our second son, was born in 1983, so the next Africa trip I couldn't leave a breastfeeding child and I felt he was still too young to leave for 2 weeks in 1984. I had also just lost my grandmother and Dad that year, and I felt like my Mom needed me. I wrote in my journal while Mike was gone for 3 weeks in 1984 that he would never GO without me again. So in 1985 it was time for me to put on my big girl panties and GO to Africa! I had to keep emphasizing the word GO because I think it is incredibly important. I've known many people throughout my life who were too scared to go, who didn't want to go, or who thought they shouldn't go. If an opportunity comes to you, prayerfully considering the idea to GO! I finally did.

I had to say goodbye to my little boys which was incredibly hard for me, but I *had* to go. I wanted to see this land that had stolen my husband's heart. My father had passed away of a sudden heart attack a year and half earlier, so my newly widowed mother, Marilyn Spaan, and my older sister, Vicki Spaan, had agreed to come to the house and keep our two boys while we were gone. I would have Gary Bohanon, our Associate Pastor, come by each morning and pick them up for school. That way, the boys' schedule remained somewhat normal and the same.

The moment I decided to go Satan began to work. Finding someone to keep both of our boys was my biggest issue and that seemed to be taken care of. My mother and sister, Vicki, had agreed to come stay at our house and keep them. They figured between the two of them, they could make it work.

The trip was planned for December. This is a busy time of year for anyone. The mission team had never gone at that time of year, but everything had worked out for that particular time. It was difficult for me because basically I had to be ready to celebrate Christmas upon my return. All gifts had to be purchased and wrapped before we left. I wanted all my Christmas decorations to be put up and ready for Christmas too. I could not stand the thought of having to come home to do all that!

The week before we were leaving I thought every mountain had been crossed. Boy was I wrong! Both Doc and Duke came down with strep throat. Doctor visits and medicine would now have to be a part of my absentee regime. My list of things the babysitter needed to know was getting longer! Perhaps it is perceptual set because we were heading there, but soon the news was showing riots in South Africa. It was occurring in Johannesburg, which was exactly where we were going to be passing through. It made me extremely apprehensive about leaving my young children.

The night before we left Mike was putting some things away in the attic. He stepped off a 2' X 4' board and his leg crashed through the ceiling to about his mid-thigh. He almost fell through the ceiling! He scraped up his leg and made a big mess in the bedroom on the floor below, not to mention a huge hole in the ceiling. That same night Oklahoma City had one of our worst infamous ice storms. Roads were simply impassible. Somehow, my mother and sister had to safely get to our house all the way across town, and we had to safely get to the airport. Truthfully, in the middle of all of this I began wondering if I should go, but we pressed on.

Twenty-one of us went on this trip, Dan and Bonnie Sheaffer, Ed & Anita Rich, Jim Elrod, Homer Bair, Lindsay Ozment, Ken Kappen, Jerry Woodie, Dave Reed, Randy Felton, Jerry & Mary Ann Gill, Jodie Usry, Paul

Odom, Claude & Robin Roberts, Ron & Jean Hawpe, Mike and I went on this trip. We left Sunday, December 1, 1985. Thankfully everyone was able to get through the ice storm to the airport safely. As we were in the air headed to Chicago, I thought the battle was over. We were on our way!

We landed on a beautiful clear Chicago sunny day. Six hours later when it was time for our flight to take-off, Chicago had begun experiencing blizzard conditions! I thought, "Are we in Oklahoma?" The same storm was happening here with snow. We almost didn't get off the ground. Our group gathered around and we prayed for our plane to be able to take off. Miraculously, there was a clearing and we were able to go. Again, I thought we were home free. Silly me!

At this point I believed the long part of the journey was over, but I was wrong. I had imagined that Europe was much farther from the U.S. than Europe is to Africa. Ha! This second leg was 14 hours instead of 9 hours. We finally landed in Johannesburg and stayed overnight. I can't tell you how wonderful it was to finally lay down in a flat position. I don't think I slept at all. Rested once again, we arrived at the airport the next day to find that Air Malawi had "wait-listed" all of us because the flight was over-booked. That wouldn't normally be a problem except there were only two flights per week into Malawi. It looked as if only a few of us would get on the flight. The remainder couldn't get there for 3 more days, as that was when the next flight was going into Lilongwe.

Right then and there our entire group again prayed for a miracle! We formed a circle and began to pray. Loudly!

Perhaps they wanted us out of the airport or perhaps they wanted to end all this evangelistic commotion, but all

30 of us got on that flight! We didn't rule out that perhaps God answers prayer! It was truly a miracle of God.

Nearing Malawi at the end of that flight, Ken Kappen was looking out the window and said, "If that's our airport, I think we just missed it." At that same moment, the plane began the steepest downward descent that I've ever experienced. It was like a kamikaze pilot! It *was* our airport and this pilot was not going to miss it, even if it meant killing us all! Though we were all petrified and worried, somehow we landed safely.

We arrived in the capital city of Lilongwe, Malawi. We then took a 30-minute bus ride to our hotel. The landscape of Malawi was nothing I had imagined. Strangely shaped acacia trees outlined the horizon and everywhere you looked. Mud huts in groups of about 15 to 20 comprised small villages along the way. Some villages couldn't be seen from the highway and yet people would appear out of small paths in the thickets. Women were walking along the road with loads on their heads and babies on their backs. It was like looking in a National Geographic. I was amazed!

I was somewhat anxious about the hotel. Mike had assured me there was a nice bathroom and bed. He was right. There were a few things he hadn't told me though. They don't have any wash clothes in Malawi. Also, the food was not what I was used to. I had brought 6 granola bars for us to snack on and realized the first day that these would have to be carefully rationed to last the entire trip! Breakfast was the only meal that even remotely seemed normal. Needless to say, I ate a big breakfast each day and squeaked by at the other meals.

Mike was right about the wonderful Malawi people. I loved them too. They were beautiful and friendly and warm. They almost always had a huge smile on their face, which seemed even bigger when their white teeth would shine from their dark skin.

The first morning I passed several local people which all said, “Morning,” to me right away. I said it back to be friendly. Later in the day people were still saying, “Morning,” to me. Since it was no longer morning, I didn’t understand why, but decided this must be their greeting – sort of like aloha or something. I didn’t find out until about 3 days later that all these people were actually saying, “Moni,” to me, which means hello in Chichewa, their native language! Ha ha! Lesson learned.

Immediately our work began. There were hours of setting up equipment, lights, musical instruments, sound equipment, and seats for the people. I knew it would be a great deal of work because Mike had described what all he did. However, some of the ones in the group who had never been on any missionary trip told me they had no idea how much work was involved. Robin Roberts told me she thought the group arrived and showed up to minister and perform. She thought the missionaries got everything ready. No way! The missionaries had definitely done many preparations beforehand, but the crusade was ours.

We had services both day and night. Genie Richmond had services for women also. Juanita Smith had services for the children. At night we had full-blown evangelistic services with the Chapelaires singing and Dan preaching. Hundreds would come forward at the altar call to accept Jesus as Savior. Seeing these beautiful people come forward was heartwarming! Only eternity will reveal the true harvest of souls! The people were instructed that if they didn’t have a church home, to attend this church which would be built at this same location.

On Sunday, we had a dedication service and the beautiful sanctuary, education wing and Pastor’s home, was dedicated to the Lord. Our interpreter, Brother Lazarus

Chakwera, was the pastor of this church. He always did a magnificent job of interpreting Pastor Sheaffer's sermons. If Pastor Sheaffer raised his right fist, Lazarus would raise his right fist, and so it went. If I remember correctly, I believe Pastor Sheaffer gave Brother Chakwera a white suit as a gift at the dedication. Brother Chakwera and his lovely wife, Monica, presented Dan and Bonnie with gifts too. I should add that all the equipment had to be brought into the church each night from the tent outside, then set up again the following day. The guys that went early to set it all up called themselves the "Roadies."

I have a vivid memory about the song the Malawi women sang during the service. It was translated to me that they were packing up their suitcases and putting it on their heads for their trip to heaven. They used their Bibles as if it were their luggage and walked around with it on their heads. Robin and I joined in the fun, but we were not as good at carrying things on our heads as these women are. They seemed thrilled that we would participate and not just watch! Even with the language barrier, it was wonderful to laugh and connect with these women and march around the church with our Bibles on our heads!

On this first trip I was so amazed at the Malawian women. They do all the work. They seed, weed and harvest the garden. They carry baskets on their heads and babies on their back. They carry the water, cook the meals, do the laundry, etc. They keep their smallest children with them by placing them in a carefully slung piece of material that is tied around their chest. When the babies need to breastfeed, they simply turn the material to the front and continue working. There were a couple of women who sang in the choir during the dedication that were nursing their infants during the song!!

Malawi's main staple is corn. They shuck the corn and dry in on a woven basket like mat in the sun. Then they pound it into a white flour meal and make what they call insema. They like insema because it is very filling. When they pound the corn, however, they pound out most of the nutrients and vitamins, but they are more concerned with feeling full than nutrition.

They also eat termites, which thrive in Africa. Yes, I'm talking about termites that eat wood and ruin houses! In Africa there were termite hills over 6 feet tall! Termites come out in the evening to mate and fly around the few light poles during certain seasons. They were everywhere! Children will huddle around that pole and grab the termites out of the air, pull of the wings and pop them into their mouths! They tell us that it tastes like a cross between salty bacon and peanuts. Some industrious women were also around the light poles and would grab the termites and throw them into a pail of water. The water would wet their wings and make it impossible for the termites to fly away. The women would later cook them for her family. It is a real delicacy and treat for them. The children also often have white faces from chewing on the baobab tree fruit. It is the same fruit from which we make cream of tartar. They tell me it tastes like a sweet-tart.

Both men and women walk everywhere they go. A few had bicycles and only the very wealthy have cars. If you do have a car, you will often have it filled with people going your direction. We were told that some charge for this luxury. There are also buses (mini-vans) which are for hire to go from place to place that cost a certain fee. These are always packed to the brim with 15-20 people. The children go to school. They are generally under a thatched roof without walls, but some of the cities do have school buildings. We could always hear them singing and doing their lessons.

One day when we drove up to set up for the crusade, all the students turned to see the car and began to chatter. We could hear the teacher reprimanding them to be quiet and pay attention! Some of the younger children (not yet school age) came to the fence to see what we were doing. Robin and I went over to talk to them. They would repeat everything that we said because they did not yet speak English. They are taught English in school. Their smiles were enough for us to communicate.

We left Lilongwe, again with problems in our reservation, which we are getting used to. We prayed and again, thankfully, we all got on the flight. After a terrible one hour shaky flight, we landed on one wheel in Blantyre! Listing heavily to one side, we finally came down on the runway. I turned and looked behind me and everyone that I could see was a strange shade of green. Jim Waldrop saw me looking at everyone so I said, "Can you believe that landing?" He replied, "That was no landing! That was a controlled crash!" Ed Rich added, "Obviously the captain has seen too many episodes of 'The Dukes of Hazard'!"

In Blantyre things were a little more normal to me. There were buildings and lots of roads. Outside the city were the same type villages as in Lilongwe. Small communities of people who needed to be near the large city for their jobs. The shopping was better here, but also more expensive. The vendors were more aggressive and would surround you. At times it was a little bit frightening.

In Blantyre the Roadies crew set up the equipment again. We had great services with hundreds filling the new building in the area called Kolakosa. The people loved the music and the singing especially the songs in Chichewa, which the Chapelaires had learned. Annette Newberry, one of our AG missionaries, had helped translate a couple more songs from English to Chichawe for them. The Chapelaires had spent hours learning the songs. It was well worth the efforts. The people loved them!

The people also loved the drums and Mike. I wrote in my journal, "I guess I have that in common with the Malawians!" We would drive up to start service and the people would chant "Mike, Mike,..." One woman told us her 9 year old son would turn over pans and beat them and chant "Mike, Mike,..." as he played. Dan and Bonnie arrived a little later than we did for service and then the people would chant "Sheaffer, Sheaffer,..." Soon Dan taught them to chant, "Jesus, Jesus, Jesus..." instead.

Hundreds were saved each night and would come forward for salvation. Many were prayed for and great deliverances occurred. Services were usually about 3 to 3 ½ hours because of all the singing, preaching, praying and altar calls. Everything except the singing had to be translated from English to Chichewa because not all of them speak English. They had a make-shift restroom with thatch around it and a hole in the ground. Many in our group utilized it, but I would not to drink too much before service and could hold it until I returned to the hotel!

The women and men do not usually sit together during service. The men sit on one side and the women and small children on the other side. There is usually an area where the school age children sit on the floor. Adults with a big stick patrol this area. If the children get out of line, they get hit with that stick. No parents seemed to mind if their child got hit because they felt it was needed to keep them quiet, and boy was it quiet!

While in Blantyre we visited their city zoo. We saw many wonderful and exotic animals. We saw them feed a lion and it was amazing how his teeth cut through the bones of his meal. We were taking pictures and looking through a medium size hole in the bars of the lion's cage. Soon, a zoo worker came and told us that we should not be that close. He told us the lion can move very fast and that area was only for employees. Man, we could have been killed, but we did get some good photos!

Later at the same zoo, Randy Felton called us over to see a cute monkey. When the group peeked into the cage, this monkey spread his legs toward us and urinated! Randy commented, “Well same to ya fellow!” It was so funny because it was as if the monkey waited until we were all looking at him and then he performed his ‘trick!’

After the crusades, Mike went to the rental car place to settle up with them for our group’s transportation. I looked out the window of my room to see my husband walking shirtless back to our hotel. I was asking him what in the world he was doing without a shirt on!?! He had a good explanation. The woman helping him kept telling him how much she liked Mike’s shirt. It was a white cotton button up shirt we had purchased as a souvenir from one of our trips to the Bahamas. It had some fancy embroidery work on it and was very pretty. Jokingly, Mike asked her if she would give him a discount if he gave her the shirt. She loved the idea and gave him a $900 discount for his $25 Bahama shirt! They both felt they got a great deal! God is good!

It was also wonderful being a part of a great missionary crusade where people were saved, healed, and filled with the Holy Spirit! I definitely wanted to go back. I, too, had fallen in love with Africa. I finally understood how important it is to GO when you are called. This was the first of my 19 trips to Africa thus far. To say the least, it was easy to GO and to…

keep smiling…

Unless the Lord builds the house,
They labor in vain who build it;
Unless the Lord guards the city,
The watchman stays awake in vain.
Psalm 127: 1 NKJV

Chapter 5 – A New House

In 1993 my husband wanted to move. He either wanted to build next door to Dan and Bonnie or move. Dan and Bonnie had built a beautiful new home in 1991. So Mike wanted a new one. We, or I should say he, began looking at new houses. He would take me to see them and I would usually say no way. I liked where we were.

The kids were all happy in their respective schools, and I wasn't sure I wanted to build or move. Two houses he liked were in the Kingswood neighborhood and I immediately said no to both. I told him I would know when it was the right house. Then in January 1994, he took me to see a house with a 'for sale' sign in front. On the way there I saw a different house – a gorgeous house, and I said, "What about that one?" He liked it too and suggested I call.

I called the number on the sign and a realtor named Cindy answered. When I asked about the house, she told me it had just been sold. Needless to say, I was disappointed. I finally found a house *I* was interested in and it's sold! I asked her to take my name and number in case it didn't go through. She hesitated and explained that the man who bought it was a physician who had been preapproved. It was all but done. Usually I'm not a pushy person, but this time I persisted. I said, "Well, we all know how these real estate things can go, so please take my number just in case!" She finally did, although she was clarifying that this particular deal was good as gold. The doctor who had purchased it, had signed a contract and was going back home simply to get the wife and kids.

I was not surprised when a few weeks later, she called and told me that the doctor had gone home to tell the family about the house and his teenage children did not want to move. They said they would rather stay where they were and live with their grandmother. Apparently the wife didn't really want to move either, so all of a sudden - it was back on the market! We arranged a showing where we could take our contractor, who would be in charge of adding the 4th bedroom. Soon we were negotiating to purchase this 5300 square foot house.

It was the most beautiful home I had ever seen. As we walked through it, I could picture my children running down the stairs to see what Santa Claus had brought! I could imagine them standing on the curved staircase for formal dances. It felt like home.

After our tour Mike and I stepped out onto the porch and he asked me what I thought. I replied, "I love this house! I never planned to like it this well!" I had mainly gone to see it to get ideas for when we would build next door to Dan and Bonnie. We had even had our gates built for our entrance, and the architect had drawn up plans for our new home. Then I went to see this house in a beautiful neighborhood on Greenbriar Chase. I loved it! I just knew in my heart this was *our* house.

The process of getting a house can give you an ulcer, yet it is so exciting! To this day, I believe the only reason we got the house was because of a God thing - our realtor was also the seller's realtor. She was negotiating for both sides. There was another buyer so we had to give them our best offer and we had to do it fast. I, naturally, wanted to lowball the offer. Mike asked me if I would be upset if the other family got the house. I said, "Yes, I'll be devastated!" He explained that we needed to give our best offer. We did and we got the house! We got the news and began thinking about moving and selling our current home. It was bittersweet! The boys would have to change schools. We would not be 3 minutes from the church anymore, and we would definitely have to get used to that. We also would not be building and moving next door to Dan and Bonnie.

Up to this point we had been planning to build a house next door to my in-laws. We had lived next door to them for over 12 years from 1982 to 1991, and been fine, so we knew this would be okay. However, when this house came into the picture, Mike showed me that he couldn't build me a house with all the accoutrements that this house had, for the same money per square foot. He believed it was a great deal even if we didn't move in. I was only looking at the gigantic price tag.

The day we signed the mortgage for a total of $940,000.00 over 30 years, I was nauseous! That wasn't the price tag. That's what the mortgage said we would end up paying after 30 years!

The day after we got the keys, we began construction on the 4th bedroom. It was a little awkward because the previous owner was still living there. He was "renting" the house for $100/day for those first few days. We had the construction crew start early the next day. We were there every morning at 7 AM which was the agreed upon time to start and stayed well into the evening. We wanted to be as loud and noisy as possible so he wouldn't stay long. Thankfully the gentleman moved out in 5 days! The construction was completed in a few short weeks and we moved out of the old house and into the new. When we moved we put our old home on the market and sold it just 3 weeks later to someone who had prequalified and wanted a quick close!

We were able to close before we had ever made one payment on the new house. I told the kids that this was a "modern day miracle!" It was June and we wouldn't have to air condition both houses, keep the pool maintained at the old house, and Mike wouldn't have to mow the lawn for both houses, not to mention making two house payments! To be kind, Mike did mow the yard the day we moved out so the new owners wouldn't have to think about that. It was sweet. Thank you Lord for blessing us with this new house!

It is so important to be grateful when things are good. Stop and thank the Lord for all the good things in your life: your health, your job, your family, your spouse, your children, your grandchildren, your house, your car, etc. – the things that really matter.

Life is good, but always remember – when you're on the mountain top, there eventually will be a valley. Yes, the valley is coming – even so…

keep smiling…

…

Chapter 6 –
Losing Mom

On a typical Saturday afternoon in September of 1996, my phone rang. It was my mother's 2nd husband, Ed Harry, calling to tell me there had been an accident. He said it was at the house Mi-mi lived in. Mother went to my Grandmother's house often and took Mi-mi places; for example, to get her hair done or to buy groceries. I kept thinking it was a car accident, and kept asking questions trying to make what he was saying fit into my preconceived idea of what he was saying. It didn't work.

There was no car wreck although a car was involved. It was an accident at my Grandmother's house. Still, my brain could not receive this news. I asked what hospital they were heading to and he said they were both gone. Gone? Gone where? I don't remember his exact words, but he kept telling me and it finally clicked that they had died.

Stunned and shaking, I called Mike to tell him that I was heading over to my grandmother's house. He said no. He didn't want me driving, and he would head home immediately to take me. I called Doc and told him. He was going to meet us there. Sesily and Duke were at the fair with some friends and wouldn't be home until later.

What do you do in an earth shattering, life-changing situation like this? What do you do when you receive the news that one of the most important people in your inner circle isn't going to be there anymore? I can only tell you what I did. When I hung up the phone from talking to Ed and then Mike, I cleaned the kitchen.

Why, you ask? I have no idea. I think I wanted to do something normal. I knew my world would never be the same.

We couldn't get there fast enough. When we arrived, we were met with television cameras, police cars, and firetrucks. I guess it isn't every day that two ladies die in the car in a hot garage. Soon my sisters arrived and I only remember a big group hug in the yard while we were all crying. We were supposed to meet for dinner that night to celebrate Steve Stephen's, Terri's husband's, birthday. We had reservations at Twelve Oaks. We had plans. This was NOT the plan.

When we arrived, Mike and Steve asked to see the "scene." The police allowed them to see it. They wouldn't let my sisters or me. We began to piece Mom's afternoon together to make sense of this nonsensical state of affairs. We didn't even know where to go. We would usually go to Mom and Ed's house, but the thought of her not being there was too much. I also had to get back to the house before the two younger kids got home from the fair. We all went our separate ways.

We found out that Mom had gone to Mi-mi's to take her lunch and help with some Saturday chores. They began doing laundry and changing the sheets on the bed. They had eaten lunch because there were a couple of plates and cups out in the sink. Earlier in the week, Mom had asked Ed to purchase some leather cleaner. The grandchildren had scuffed up the back of the two front seat chairs with their shoes and Mom wanted to get it off. Mom drove a Jaguar XJS. We often teased her about being the "Little Old Lady from Pasadena." Not many 67 year olds drive a sporty car like that.

Mike later told me that Mom was found sitting in the back seat, behind the driver seat, with the leather cleaner and a rag in her hands. Mi-mi was sitting in the front passenger seat in her robe. Her walker was near the garage door entrance to the house. The garage door opener was beneath Mi-mi's robe in between the center console and the passenger seat. The third and final load of laundry was still in the dryer. There were a few of Mi-mi's blouses hung up to air dry.

We determined that Mi-mi must have followed Mom out to the garage. It was mid-September in Oklahoma so it was hot - Oklahoma muggy 90 degrees hot! We assumed they wanted to turn on the air-conditioning for just a few minutes to cool off. The police told us, it probably didn't take much more than a few minutes to kill them both. There were several reasons for this. Mom's Jaguar XJS had a 12 cylinder engine, a huge engine. The garage was built in the 1940's when they were built to be air tight. The combination made it fatal. Now, my beautiful 67 year old Mom and my 94 year old Grandmother were both gone. It was unbelievable.

A Meals-On-Wheels delivery person who came twice each week, was familiar with Mi-mi and was concerned when the front door was open, yet she didn't answer. Fortunately the screen door wasn't locked, so she came in, noticed how smoky the house was, called Mi-mi's name, but there was no answer. She followed the smoke and found them in the car. It was too late.

I was so incredibly sad when my dad died, but mom?!? She was my best friend and confidante. Who would I go to in times of need? Who would I call to tell funny stories to about my kids? Who was going to fill my love tank? To say I was devastated is again, an understatement. I was overcome with grief. I was trying to be strong for my family, but inside I was in shock. I couldn't really speak. There was nothing to say.

When we got home that evening, Duke had already been told by Doc. Duke told me later that he began to cry, so he just left the house and started walking. We were there a little while when Sesily was brought home by the family she went to the fair with. When she came in, we all stood up and met her in the kitchen. We tried to gently tell her that her "Mom-o" was gone.

She immediately started crying and said, "She was so nice!" It struck me that a child goes straight to the heart of the matter. Mom *was* nice. It was worth crying over. When she said that, we all had a big group hug and we were all crying even harder with her sweet sentiment. In my heart of hearts I knew things would never be the same again. My mother was my rock, my touchstone. Without that foundation, I wasn't sure what would happen next. I prayed for Jesus to help me. The only thing I knew to do was to...

keep smiling...

Chapter 7 – I Saw It Coming

My situation is not unlike yours. We all can find ourselves in a mess. I thought I had been in the worst mess of my life just a few short years before when I had lost my mom. However, life socked me in the gut once again. My middle son, Duke, told Mike and I that he was gay. Being a fundamentalist Assembly of God family and attending a church, where homosexuals are told quite frequently they are going to hell, this was especially excruciating news. It doesn't get much worse than that or so I thought. I thought I was well-acquainted with pain. I had lost both parents, all of my grandparents, and seriously thought I had been through the worst of it.

The roller coaster of life was not finished with me. This was a new turn. It's a long story that I won't go into the details, but my sister, Duke's Aunt Vicki, had a hand in telling us. Duke felt betrayed and was absolutely furious with her. It took many years for them to rebuild their relationship.

Now I could stop here and write an entire book on dealing with this new information. I could tell you so many things I learned during those painful times, but just know that God is good. It is during these times that we have to stay with God. We often want to run away from Him and feel as if He has failed us.

I like to think of a young child who isn't getting his way. They cry, scream, kick, and basically act terrible because they aren't getting their way. They sometimes run away from the parent that isn't doing exactly what they want. In most cases, the parent just stands by and watches. They aren't impressed by this valiant show of will. Parents are generally waiting for the tantrum to be over before they respond. I believe God does the same thing. He allows us to "get it all out" before he answers. Some call this "the In-Between Time." As I read Matt Nelson's book about this years later, I recognized it. This is where I was. I wanted things to be different. I wanted God to make things right again. I was in the desert and I didn't like it there.

I cried. I prayed. I read books on how to handle this. I cried some more. I prayed some more. I called on God to "fix" my son. I did everything I knew to do. Notice how all those things start with "I." Finally, after months of this, "I" turned it all over to God.

God had been so patient, so loving, so compassionate and caring with me during this period. He just waited patiently for me to come to terms with it. He loved me unconditionally even as I was screaming for him to do something!!! I was somewhat like Lieutenant Dan in the movie Forest Gump. God was tolerant and walked alongside of me as a longsuffering comrade in a battle that I did not know how to win. God did not judge me as I threw my tantrum of tears and pleas. He did not push me out. He stayed quiet and uncomplaining by my side. After weeks of longing for an answer from the Lord, in one of my prayers, I finally got quiet. Instead of praying and telling God what I wanted Him to do, I fell silent.

I had never thought of silence as prayerful. Previously in my prayer time, I was always talking, asking, and reminding the Lord of everything He had promised. Now I was at a place where I had nothing else to say. I had no words left. I had asked for change, yet God was silent. I finally became silent myself.

> *In the silence I truly felt*
> *the Lord tell me what I needed to do –*
> *"Love him."*

I burst into tears. *"By **this**...shall all men know that you are my disciples," John 13:35,* is now one of my favorite scriptures. It wasn't one of my favorites until I traveled this road. To love my son would be the easiest thing Jesus had ever asked me to do!

That was too easy. That was too simple. All the fear and hopelessness faded into the background. This was a task that I could do! I love my middle son so very much. I always have. He is smart, intelligent, a risk taker, thoughtful, and fun! So loving Duke comes easily to me. Granted, he can be curt and if you ever get into a verbal altercation with him, his words can hurt and cut like a knife, when he wants to injure. If Duke is mad at you, he is like trying to love a porcupine! However, when he's sweet, he is the absolute best!

The funny thing is my husband and I had always – since his toddler years - suspected he was gay. As early as his second birthday, we saw it. My mom, his grandmother, had said to me, "If this child turns out to be gay, I'll know it was hereditary." I was furious! No one wants to hear that their child might be gay! -Let alone that someone else sees what you see.

It's funny even writing that now. Because all these many years later, her words now give me peace. Her words now reassure me that I didn't cause it. I believe he was born this way. Some say that it is a choice – especially those in the church. Duke assures me that if he had any choice, it would not be this one.

You may close this book and disagree with me, but I did not come here to disagree. I wrote this to simply explain *my* journey. My story of an exceedingly challenging season in my life. I actually believe it may have been the beginning of the undoing of my marriage. It was also a point where my prayers seemed futile and unanswered.

> *Blessed is the man who trusts me, God,*
> *the woman who sticks with God.*
> *They're like trees replanted in Eden,*
> *putting down roots near the rivers –*
> *Never a worry through the hottest summers,*
> *Never dropping a leaf, Serene and calm through*
> *droughts, bearing fresh fruit every season.*
> *Jeremiah 17:7-8 MSG*

A different version says it like this:

> *Blessed is the man who trusts in the Lord,*
> *And whose hope is the Lord.*
> *For he shall be like a tree planted by the waters,*
> *Which spreads out its roots by the river,*
> *And will not fear when heat comes;*
> *But its leaf will be green,*
> *And will not be anxious in the year of drought,*
> *Nor will cease from yielding fruit.*
> *Jeremiah 17:7-8 NKJV*

Perhaps you find yourself in a period where you are questioning whether God hears your cries. Perhaps you are going through a difficult trial. Perhaps you have just discovered that your child is gay. Lay it all at the feet of Jesus. Hand all your worries, disappointments, and fears over to Him. We are told to cast our cares on him. Some synonyms for cast are: hurl, throw, fling, or toss. That means to cast with gusto! Give it to Him! Hurl it to Jesus! Like an angry kid throwing something at mom and dad's feet when they don't get their way. Jesus can take it! He told us to do this!!!

However, Duke telling us he was gay was a Catch 22. I was so thankful that he could trust us with his most intimate and private thoughts. I was also disappointed on many levels. I was saddened because I knew that meant he would probably not have children of his own. I knew this would be a difficult and problematic road to travel especially in our church's circles. I knew he would be shunned by some, because I also immediately knew, or thought I knew, how the church would react. I had very little faith in my fellow Christ followers. Some would absolutely shine and come through. Others stepped way back, not wanting to get our "cooties." lol

This brings up why we, as Christ followers, always seem to care so much about what the church thinks. We should be more concerned about what Jesus thinks! That, however, is easier said than done. We *should* look at the fact that in the Bible, Jesus almost always chose to be with the outcasts, the people religion had ostracized. When Jesus asked the woman at the well, who was a known Samaritan for some water, He knew the religious people wouldn't approve. That's why He did it! He was telling us right there that he wants the outsider, the social pariah, and the castaway. He invites them in and offers His best living water!

In the beginning when Mike and I found out, we didn't discuss it much together. It was too painful. I think we both thought if we didn't discuss it, it would go away. I mentioned seeing a counselor and his response was that *we* were not the ones with a problem. He offered to pay for Duke to go. We certainly didn't tell any of our friends what we were going through. That took years. Looking back, I believe this situation took a real toll on our marriage. This is when deeply rooted problems began. Please know, I am certainly not blaming Duke! I am blaming our inability as a couple, to come together to grieve and cope openly with what was happening in our family.

I also felt Mike possibly took it as a blow to his masculinity. I think he felt somehow responsible. He was always closer to our oldest son, Doc. He spent more time with Doc. He and Doc had sports to discuss. They enjoyed playing them and watching them. Duke was generally left out of those conversations. Duke was also left out of watching the sports on television and discussing what was being watched. In the early years Mike tried to include him, but to no avail. Therefore, Duke spent most of his time with me.

He liked music and playing piano like I do. He was in Honor Choir and loved to sing. He was never good at sports. If he tried to play on the driveway, Doc would beat him so savagely that it was not fun for him at all! I do think Doc's abilities and athletic prowess made Duke feel like a failure in any sport he tried. Maybe it was Doc's fault – in fact, let's blame him! lol

Maybe it was no one's fault. One time, when we were on a mission trip in Africa, Becky and Dan Garland were keeping our kids and took Duke to play in one of his basketball games. She said he was floating down the court like a ballerina! I knew exactly what she meant because I saw it during each and every game. He could have cared less about the game, but was very interested in his dance moves getting down the court!

Duke had also wanted Sweet Secrets toys for his 2nd birthday. This was an unusual request but I tried to not put too much weight into a two year old's requests. He wanted a purse like Amanda Beckley for Christmas when he was three. These were indicators.

He loved to swim and snow ski, but otherwise had no inkling for sports. We tried. We put him on a t-ball team at 4 years old. He could have cared less. He played soccer at 5. He loved socializing on the bench much more than the games. We have video of him talking nonstop on the bench and barely running on the field. He played basketball at 6. He floated down the court. He asked to take dancing lessons at around this time and I put him in dance class. He was bullied about it at school and so that didn't last long. We had him go out for football in junior high. We tried everything we could think of to make him more masculine.

He was more masculine than his brother in some ways. We had noticed Duke wasn't scared of the wolf in a movie called, "The Never Ending Story," that terrified Doc. We pounced on this. We let him watch the movie, 'Ghostbusters" at 4 years old because it wasn't feminine. Doc was scared to watch it. We bought him every toy they sold for Ghostbusters! We were thrilled that he wanted something that wasn't a girl's toy. To this day, Duke loves scary movies and books. I feel responsible. Ha! We had such a positive reaction to him watching these, that it makes sense.

The friends that Duke would invite over were also somewhat feminine, except for a few. Mike and I had some conversations where we expressed the possibility that he might be gay. We always laughed it off with, "This is just a phase."

When Duke was in the 8th grade, Mike discovered a magazine with pictures of nude men. He confronted Duke, and Duke admitted it was his. He even told his dad he thought he was gay. I found out years later that in another conversation Mike told him not to say anything to me. He said to Duke, "This will kill your mom, so don't tell her." He didn't, until he was 21 in 2004. His life was spiraling out of control. He couldn't contain this secret any longer. He decided to let the chips fall where they may.

Looking back, I'm sad that Duke had to grapple with his sexuality and his Christianity alone. I know he prayed for years as he puts it, to "Pray the gay away!" I didn't know what to do and it also sent me to my knees. I had to pray like I had never prayed before. I wanted and asked God to fix it for me. My Assembly of God-taught heart didn't want a child of mine to be in a category listed as sin. I didn't want a gay son. I wanted Duke to have a wife and children. I didn't want him to be faced with a life of being rejected.

I knew that if certain people in the church knew this about my son, he would no longer be accepted. I'm telling you this because looking back, I was wrong. There were so many Christian friends who did accept him – just as he was! They loved him with no judgment right alongside of me and still do. It has been a tremendous blessing in my life and his. Thank you Lord for people who are real and believe and do what the Good Book says!

Now that I had finally come to understand that my part was to simply love Duke, I could do exactly what God had done for me. Like God I could be patient, loving, and caring for him. I could just walk patiently beside him as he confronted new struggles. I could love him unconditionally. I could spend nonjudgmental time with Duke and walk alongside of him as a tolerant and accommodating comrade in a battle that I did not know how to win. I could practice not judging Duke or the situations that were to surely come. I would not push him away, but stay uncomplaining and quiet by his side. I could be Jesus in this circumstance. Could I do it?

With effort, Duke and I did work through this on our own time. Duke continued to struggle to connect with his dad, which was the norm. Mike made little effort to get along or begin a new journey with this knowledge. Mike was cordial yet cold to Duke. Therefore, Duke generally stayed away from the family and the church. That's how he coped. Duke and I started by talking on the phone. That's how we reconnected, and over time we rebuilt our relationship. I was no longer judging. I was loving. Duke could tell. I remembered the scripture in Romans 2:4 that says it's the goodness of God that calls men to repentance:

> *Are you [actually] unaware or ignorant [of the fact] that God's kindness leads you to repentance. Romans 2:4 AMP*

I truly learned to pray and depend on God during these days. I learned to be quiet after my prayers. It is in this silence that I can hear God. I am quiet, so that God has room and opportunity to speak to me. Most importantly, I learned to give the outcome to the Lord. Duke and I made it through our darkest days and came out stronger than ever and that alone makes me want to...

keep smiling...

Wait on the Lord:
be of good courage,
and He shall strengthen thine heart:
wait, I say, on the Lord.
Psalm 27:14 KJV

Chapter 8 – Waiting

Somewhere at the end of 2005 and the beginning of 2006, I completely stopped trusting my husband. I knew something was going on. I knew we were no long "one." There really is something to the scripture that the two become one, because I knew immediately when we weren't. I don't say that lightly, because we continued to have great sex throughout this period. Yet, something was different. I just couldn't put my finger on it. I couldn't have told you exactly what was wrong, I just knew *something* was different.

Let me give a little background to provide a better understanding of the situation. On Valentine's Day 2006, my husband and I gave sweet Valentine cards to one another.

My card to Mike said:

I Love You More Than Ever! On the inside it said: For all the loving things you do…For all the dreams you made come true…For sharing life, for being you…I love you more than ever.

Happy Valentine's Day.
I Love You,
Sandy

I also included a letter for him that said:

Dear Mike,

Well, it is really hard to believe that we are looking at another Valentine's Day. The first Valentine's Day I spent with you, I was 15 years old – the age of our daughter. It was 1972 – 34 years ago – which makes this the 35th Valentine together. My how the years have flown.

I still feel the same way I did back then. I feel like I still have my whole life ahead of me even though I know I don't. I feel young even though I know that I'm not. I feel like you are the most important person in my life and that is the one thing that is the same – truly. I love you more now than I did then. But only because I know better your true worth and value. I know what a wonderful human being you are.

I know you work a lot and I hate that, but I love how successful you are. I hate the long hours you put in, but I love how well you provide for your family. I hate you getting up at 5:45 AM every morning to work out, but I love your physic and what a handsome man you are. I hate you being gone in the evenings, but I love your dramas and CD's and things that have such an impact on people's eternal life. I hate you leaving us and traveling to Africa to preach and build tabernacles, but I am so proud of your commitment to God and to doing what He has commanded us – to go into all the world and preach the gospel.

I know I can be difficult to live with sometimes but even in those times, I think you know how much I love you. You mean more to me than words could ever really say. You truly are my soul mate. I am so fortunate to have found you and that you have stayed by my side throughout this magnificent journey. Through 35 Valentine's Days, through 29 and a half years of marriage, through the births and lives of our three wonderful children and now our grandson (isn't he precious?), it has been great. Of course, there have been difficult times. Those difficult times have only made the good times seem better. I don't think I would change a thing. I look through my scrapbooks and I feel so blessed that this is MY life and that you have been willing to spend it with me.

Happy Valentine's Day! I love you,
Sandy

Mike's card to me said:

For the beautiful woman who shares my life. On the inside it said: … On Valentine's Day, find new ways to tell her how perfect she is for you – how perfectly she fits into your arms, your heart, your life…Find new ways to tell her how much she means to you – how much you admire her, respect her, need her, want her… Find new ways to tell her you care, as you share smiles or sadness, as you listen, as you touch and kiss and embrace…One way or another, I've told myself these things, and today, I want to share them with you. Because more than anything, I want you to know how much I love you…sometimes more than I can say.

Happy Valentine's Day.
I Love You!
Mike

He also included a letter that read:

Sandy,

HAPPY VALENTINE'S DAY! I am so sorry you're feeling under the weather. I want you to know how much I love you, admire you, appreciate you and respect you. You are truly a wonderful woman. As a wife, you are beyond compare. As a mother, there is none more diligent. As a confidant, none are wiser. As a lover, you should be in the movies. And as a friend, you are simply the best! Thank you for being mine. You mean more to me than you will ever know and I will always love you.

Happy, Happy Valentine's Day.
Mike

I put these two cards here in the book to show we did have genuine and deep feelings for one another.

Don't get me wrong, it was not a good time in our 35 years. I knew something had changed. We had had other times in our relationship where we grew apart, yet always came back together with time spent one on one. I hoped that was what was happening. I think most relationships experience this. We had our busy lives with church work and the lives of our three children keeping us apart - that's what I was trusting it was. I kept telling myself it was the fact *he* was so busy.

Beginning here, some is in the present tense because many of these paragraphs are from my journals:

*Lately he has been coming home late and leaving early, and doing things that he thinks I don't know about or notice. He has been acting strange and doing strange things. Somewhere in the past few months, I decided he thinks I'm gullible and am oblivious to what he's doing. He is a terrible liar! What's crazy is that he thinks he's good at it. He's not, and I am certain he is lying to me. I know he has had drama practice, an Africa trip to plan, year-end accounting duties, etc. He is a busy guy, *but* he also doesn't tell me everything. After we read the cards, Mike actually had tears in his eyes and said that I was "the winner" because my letter was better. I had to agree with him. We spent Valentine's Day with Sesily at Grandy's. How romantic! How do we keep this relationship where it needs to be?!? I'm kidding, only I am not kidding. I truly didn't mind because we had drama rehearsal for the upcoming Easter pageant.

A few days after Valentine's Day, Mike got up at 4:30 AM supposedly to see Terry Williams off at the airport for their upcoming Africa trip. He didn't come home until 7:30 AM. That was odd. He claimed he went to church and worked. I knew he was lying. For some reason, this really upset me. I began crying which I rarely do, and told him I'm used to the dregs of his time, and I'm not even getting that anymore. Mike was his typical emotionally-unavailable self! Later I was still furious. However, now he was really trying to be nice and spend time with me, to make up for it. He certainly doesn't want me upset. He packed. I just laid on the bed and didn't help at all. I just couldn't. Usually I helped him, but I just watched him pack. Mike had decided this trip would be a guy's only trip.

The next day was Sunday. Mike left the house @ 2:45 PM and I soon followed. I sat in the apartment parking lot watching the church until 3:40 and he never came to church. I knew he wouldn't. I knew he never went to Walmart for stuff for the missionary, which is where he claimed he was going. All I know to do is to pray for the Lord to help me to do this. I have to be strong. I don't really want to know, but God help me, I have to know.

There were several things that have lead me to make this decision. At church a couple of weeks ago Barbara Eidson, the church secretary, even said something about him having a girlfriend. I had my suspicions and I felt she was trying to help me, so I became nosier. On Friday, January 27, when I went to work out, I drove by church (which is where he said he was going). I left @ 7:25 AM and @ 8:25 AM I drove by church and he still wasn't there. What was he doing for over an hour? Another time he called from his car phone and said he was at the church. He didn't know I can tell the difference between his normal cell phone and when he's in the car. He lied to me.

On February 2, he said he had been golfing. He was very late and claimed he was stuck @ 74th and Penn due to a wreck there. He went @ 12:30 and was probably through @ 4:30. This was almost 6. When I pressed him he made up a story about how he was going to go to the health food store but didn't because of the wreck. It was weird and I didn't believe him. I was definitely seeing a pattern.

On Wednesday February 1, Gary Bohanon called and Mike wasn't at church (this was about 3:15). I called and Mike acted to me like he was at church. He never said otherwise. He didn't know that I knew he wasn't there. On January 26, the day before I drove by church and checked up on him, Mike and I took Sesily to Arby's for a fast lunch. She had a string on her shirt and I asked Mike to get out his clippers and clip it. When he did, a Viagra fell out of his pocket. That is probably the moment I knew for sure that he was having an affair and that it was, obviously, sexual.

My heart began to beat at an absurd rate. My eyes were darting around the room which was now spinning. I was praying to myself that neither Mike nor Sesily notice my peculiar behavior. They didn't seem to. I quickly cleared the table and said we needed to be on our way. Mike kissed us both goodbye and was off. He seemed glad that lunch was cut short – I now knew why. He was going to see *her* – whoever this "her" was! He gave me time to get Sesily to school and about 10 minutes later called. He told me what it was and said he didn't want Ses to see and ask questions. He said he liked to take Viagra to "feel bigger." I knew he was lying. I knew this was just his cover story. Now I'm wondering why he's carrying Viagra to work???? I already know the answer. Is it someone at work or perhaps drama practice? He had drama that night.

Now for a little history on how I first began not trusting him and why it was so easy to quit trusting him again. In January or February of 2004, Mike and I were sitting in a theatre waiting for '*Cold Mountain*' to come on and his phone rang. It was a woman from the church.

I considered her a friend. Immediately I recognized her voice, and I could hear her ask if this was a bad time. Mike moved the phone to the opposite ear, I guess thinking that would keep me from hearing their conversation. They talked for a couple of minutes and hung up. He didn't know I could hear everything, including the voice of who it was. I asked who it was and he said it was his uncle. He lied to my face again. I was dumbfounded! -So much so that I couldn't yet confront him about all these lies. I had to decide what to do and how to do it. That night was a party for Eddie Loomis @ the church. I watched as Mike went to get some dessert and I saw him go up real close behind this woman and hit the back of her knee with his. They giggled and talked for a moment, and then he moved on.

All that wouldn't be that weird except a few years earlier (I'm sure I could find when in my journals) I went to church and Barb said Mike was in the sanctuary. I went over there and couldn't find him. I went to Dan's waiting room and it was locked. That was odd. I thought I heard something going on and when I knocked, there was shuffling around. Soon, there he was, opening the door, trying to get me to not go in there. He tried to come out into the hall and close the door behind him. He was acting very peculiar. I pushed past him and thought I saw a shadow in Bon's room so I walked in there and was suddenly face to face in the dark with this woman I "thought was my friend." My heart sank.

Oh, they had their "story" ready for me. Supposedly they were there discussing her daughter's financial woes and needs from the church. If it had actually been that, Mike would have taken care of it from his office, where the checkbook is nearby. I stewed on it for a day or two. When I confronted Mike about the previous phone call, he said they were planning me a birthday party. Remember this is in January and my birthday is in July - an awfully long time to plan. I threatened to call her and did. She said the exact same thing - almost word for word. Both were too rehearsed. It seemed like a story they had decided to tell together. I didn't believe either one. She also said, "Don't provide him with any answers." I wondered, "What does that mean?" My thoughts are all over the place.*

Back to writing in the past tense:

Our relationship had gotten so much worse since last summer. I also need to insert that way back in 1989 Mike had been having inappropriately long phone conversations with another church lady. I caught him going to her place of work and talking to her on the phone. She got stranded in a snow storm and called Mike to pick her up. He was gone for 2 ½ hours which was way over the time it would have taken him to go help her. I was done. I actually told him I wanted a divorce. He took my hands with my two large rings and began hitting his own face with my hands!!! He cut up his face and my hands. I refused to sing at church that morning with the woman he'd been calling.

The following day we had a trip planned to Palm Springs. I wasn't going to go, but he cried – *real* tears - and begged me to go so we could work on our marriage. I relented and went, and we did just that. I truly felt we had worked it out. I guess God was helping us because almost as soon as we returned to OKC, the woman's unknowing husband had been transferred to Chicago and within two more weeks, they were gone. God is good. Snap! She is not only out of my singing group, the Sweet Inspirations, and the church, but they have moved completely out of the state.

I should add that I truly did trust him again, and even got pregnant the following year because Mike was being so loving and attentive. Life was good. Here is the trouble, however. When you have lost someone's trust, it is particularly easy to lose it again. As soon as I overheard that phone call in 2004 (page 74), my trust evaporated in an instant. Every time he left the house or got a phone call, I presumed he was going to see someone or was talking to someone. This time I was more cynical. I decided to hire a private investigator.

I felt guilty that I didn't trust him. One meme says, "Trust takes years to earn and seconds to lose." I had sincerely hoped he was being faithful, but there was a wedge between us. Last but not least, Travis and Rachel saw him on a pay phone at 12th and Santa Fe on Friday, September 16, 2005, in the morning. He also had bought another cell phone. It's another number that I don't know and I don't get a bill for – huge red flag! Why would you need to keep a phone number from your wife if it's on the up and up? Then on February 8 a man called my cell and said Mike was coming to see a car at 3 or so when he got off work. Now I thought it was possible he was getting a different car. Perhaps I was paranoid. All this had made me this way. I didn't sleep well because Mike gets up during the night and creeps around. I would act asleep. I knew something was going on and I had to know what it was. The perfect time to find out was while he was gone. Help me Lord!

On February 23, 2006, I wrote in my journal: "I took the kids to school then fasted lunch. I went to see Dr. Chambers. She's so nice but I wouldn't go if I didn't need that prescription. I heard from Mike – they put up a tabernacle today. He said it was a day of firsts. 1st tabernacle in Burundi, 1st missions group, etc. I wanted to tell him it was a day of firsts for me too, because today I met with the Private Investigator. It was scary and I was shaking. He seems okay. He told me that there is a 98% chance he is having an affair. He said if Mike is, he will catch him. He claimed that by the time the wife calls him, they just want proof. I told him that my prayer is that I would be one of those 2% and then I could trust him again.

I had to give him a picture of Mike and tell him tag numbers of his cars. The PI knew who we were and had even been to our dramas. He was shocked to learn that he would be following the man who portrayed Jesus! I could see the disappointment on his face.

When I got home, I cleaned out our closet. I keep hoping to find something with "her" name on it or some indicator of what is going on. I found nothing. I helped Sesily study for 4 tests. Mike called again this evening. He is being sweeter than ever. It's a fake kind of 'sweeter.' I think it is to cover up what he's doing. Maybe I'm wrong about all of this. I hope so."

I kept trying to be hopeful that this was not true. I prayed so. However, all this sugary sweetness from him was so unnatural. It was sort of sickening. He was definitely trying to hide something. It was like he was trying to keep me content and happy. He had never before cared if I was content and happy. He certainly hadn't had to work at it so much. It made me know that he was covering for something.

All of this make me remember back in March of 1999 when Mike had said to me, "It's time to lose weight and get a new hairdo." I mean, what loving husband says that? Why not say, "Let's go on a walk together?" After he said this, for the first time in my journal I wrote that I was sick of Mike. He had always been very shallow and only into what I looked like.

Maybe he had grown tired of me being a little overweight. All of this made me wonder.

The Lord provided me a scripture from Psalm 27:14:

Wait on the Lord:
Be of good courage,
And he shall strengthen thine heart:
Wait, I say, on the Lord.
Psalm 27:14 KJV

I had been praying so diligently for God's help. He had given me such guidance. I had never needed God so much in my life. I always thought I was close to Him, and I realize now I wasn't. I'm learning through all of this and drawing closer to Him every day. I'm also learning that sometimes when it is the hardest, we have to be hopeful and…

keep smiling…

… here I am, your invited guest—
it's incredible!
I enter your house; here I am,
prostrate in your inner sanctum,
Waiting for directions
to get me safely through enemy lines.
Psalm 5:7-8 MSG

Chapter 9 –
Still Waiting

This chapter will be mainly journal entries to explain what was happening during these days so it may vacillate between past and present tense:

*I didn't sleep well last night. My heart goes 90 miles per hour when I think of this whole deal. I have to know. I think I know that there is something going on. Mike called me @ 10 AM yesterday and again at 9 PM. At 9 PM he said his cell phone was almost out of time. That's weird because he said yesterday they were getting new sim cards. I know he didn't call his mom or the office because I spoke with them. I wondered on Wednesday when he had called so often if he were doing that to "cover" his calls to someone else. If he's on the phone a lot and someone tells me – then I will think he was on the phone with me. We never talked very long except one conversation on Wednesday for about 10 minutes. I remember thinking why is he calling just to tell me this? Hopefully I'm just paranoid but the PI didn't think so. Lord, help me to find out so I can have peace. If he is, I want to know. If he isn't, I want to trust him again and put this behind me.

While Mike was gone to Africa on Saturday, February 25, 2006, I slept until 9 AM then got up and washed my hair. I went to Java Dave's with Ses & Duke. I received a weird call for Mike on *my* phone. I asked who was calling and she said, "Satin." It was a sultry sounding woman and all I could think of was like a stripper. It was weird. I told the kids what she'd said. Duke called her back. Satin answered and said it was some apartments in Del City and she had a wrong number, which led to a discussion on fidelity. It got us talking. Duke said he has been suspicious about dad since I told him about Mike on a pay phone (pg 77). Duke feels I have reasons to be suspicious. I tried to downplay it to Ses. I didn't want her to think anything bad about her dad. I gave Duke "the look" so he would stop talking about it. I also got our mobile phone bill and it was fine, but if he has another cell phone he'd be using that. I'm just confused and want to know. Duke said he'd snoop for me. I was sort of glad this came up because I don't want the kids to be blindsided if this turns out to be a real affair. I went to Penn Square with Ses and Duke. We found a lot. We came back here and got Ses ready for her basketball banquet. She looked great. She went with Levi. I babysat Trip and wrote:

I heard from Mike at 10 AM. He kept saying he had to go because he wasn't sure how much time he had left on his cell phone. Not so weird, but at 10:15 AM Ses wanted to ask him a question. We began calling and it was busy until 10:35. Hmmm, just as I thought… When Ses asked him who he was talking to, he first said, "I have no idea." Then a couple of minutes later he rattled off, "Bill Moore, Terry Williams and the phone card people." Only it would have been 6:30 PM on a Saturday night. I've been to Burundi and things close up early, so I don't believe him. I think he called whoever he is having an affair with and talked for several minutes. I've been thinking that's why he's calling all the time – to cover the fact that he's calling someone else so much. He has his own room for the first time *ever*, so he can make those calls without anyone else hearing.

Duke and I talked about all this later on without Sesily. Duke doesn't know I've already hired a private investigator. Man, this is getting wilder by the day but I'm at peace because the Bible says, "Be sure your sins will find you out." Funny, I've always thought of that scripture as a disciplinary tool to keep us in line. I've never thought of that scripture as a promise. Until now.

Feb. 27, 2006: Mike called at 7:15 AM. I'm thinking he has never called me this much. He never has much to say. I had to call him at 4 PM yesterday (midnight his time) to find out how to get sound on. He said this morning he'd hoped he "wasn't rude to me." He was very abrupt, bordering on rude and, hey, he was in a dead sleep. He said his back hurts. He's icing it. This was also weird because Mike has never been a really thoughtful man who worried if he was rude to someone or not, especially me or the kids! Ha!

I told him Dennis did good in Sunday School class. Dan preached great and said, "I'm ba-a-ack!" He ran the aisles! It was great! The choir did "Look for Me," with me, Tracy and Daniel as a trio. My voice was practically gone as usual.

Wednesday, March 1, 2006: I just got off the phone with Mike *again* from Africa. He is being *so* sweet and loving. He is either turning over a new leaf of being sweet or he is definitely trying to cover his cheating tracks! Ha! Maybe I'm wrong. I hope so. I pray so. Yesterday, I looked over the mobile telephone bill – there were 4 dates I'd written down to see who he was talking to on the phone. None of the times were on the bill, which means I am correct about a second mobile phone. One of the calls he claimed to be talking to his sister, but it didn't show a call at all. He told me his car needed a different phone. When I asked the number, he had claimed it was the same.

There are definitely red flags everywhere. I'm so glad things are already in the works. I have to know. I checked the dates I saw him on the phone and he said he was talking to his sister. I saw him in my rear view mirror. He was flirting and he was surprised I noticed! Give me a break. He's been flirting with me for 35 years so I should know it well; all dates - no call. Jesus, reveal what needs to be revealed.

I'm excited and scared to know the truth but I *have* to know the truth and I want to know. At the airport in baggage claim, he loudly announced to everyone, "I'm going home to have sex with my wife!" He wanted all of those people to think that he was in love with me. Funny thing is that he never had to worry about what they thought before. Why now? I am afraid I know. We all really missed him! The PI will follow him tomorrow morning, so I'll know something soon.

On Saturday, the PI followed Mike to church, but he was only there about 10 minutes. He went north on Shields to I-240, then east. That's where the PI lost him. He said Mike was speeding. That's unusual. My questions weren't answered, but he lied, He told me he was there the entire time. The PI missed the best opportunity. I should mention that twice this weekend, Mike cried. Once at the end of the movie, "*16 Blocks*" about how people can change. Then again Sunday AM talking to me about Burundi and the next crusade. It's weird. I know he is jet-lagged from his trip, but it's strange. What is he crying about? The guilt? The fact that everyone could find out about his infidelity?

I honestly feel he can't stand me. I am surprised that I'm not more upset by all this. It's weird – like I already know. My heart is so callused. When I look up the word callus, it means hardening over a wound. I know I am wounded from his previous infidelities. I have little feeling for him. At times I can't stand him. I just need proof now. Help me Lord! The PI and I talked about when would be the best time to follow him again and decided this week. *End journal entries.*

To say the least, it was a long week. I had to remind myself to never doubt. Whatever was going to happen was exactly what God had for me. I had to trust the end result to Him. I had done all I knew to do. I had prayed. I had Christian friends praying with me. I hadn't told them what was happening; I just asked for their prayers. I was hoping we could get counseling and move forward with no one knowing we had some issues. I know some of you who are reading may be going through the same thing. Perhaps your story is different, yet you're still in a time of waiting to see how your story will proceed. Just know that God is with you every step of the way. It may feel like you are all alone and that God has forsaken you. Let me assure you, He hasn't.

I've been told when God closes a door He opens a window… What they forget to tell you is that it is hell in the hallway. Your heart may be on the floor in a million pieces, but just hold on. Wait. The word 'wait' means staying in a place of expectation. It means to be ready and available. I personally don't like waiting. Patience is NOT one of my virtues. I want what I want and I want it now. If you are in a period of waiting, turn to the Lord. Pray for patience. Pray for Him to be with you and attend to your needs as you wait. It may be a short wait, but it may be a long wait. God doesn't work on our time table. Even in the waiting, remember to…

keep smiling…

Chapter 10 –
Sometimes God Closes a Door

I woke up early on Wednesday, March 8, 2006, and shockingly Mike apologized for not having any time for me! It's like he knows I know. Something is different and he is trying his best to be extremely sweet and thoughtful. He thinks I haven't noticed his actions before, but now wants to try and get along so I won't be suspicious. Oops, too late! Mike, Doc, Rachel, Travis and I ate at Java Dave's. A lady from church came in. Mike sure acted strange when I invited her to sit with us. He even said angrily under his breath through clenched teeth, "Don't ask her to sit with us." I insisted and got up to get her a chair. I wrote in the back of my journal that day, "Could it be her?" We had piano lessons. I took Ses to a private lesson for the upcoming pom pon try-outs. Mike stayed at church until well after 10 PM – weird. He claimed it was for drama – uh huh, I believe you, you liar! Insert an eye roll here! lol

We had a big argument on Friday. Mike and I went to our Sunday School class - the Young Marrieds' Chili Cook-off. When we got in the car, he threatened me and said with gritted teeth, "You better not leave tonight like you did last time." I said in a high register voice, "Ooh, I'm scared of you," taunting him. I was livid. The evening was fun and I enjoyed it, in spite of

Mike being there. I didn't sit by him at all or speak to him the entire evening. It has gotten to the point that I almost can't stand being near him. I prayed, "Help me Lord to quit feeling this way. Help me God to find out the truth so I can have some peace because if he's not, we need to work on our marriage."

I didn't know it yet, but my prayers were about to be answered.

I found out from the PI that my husband was having an affair with a gal that stood beside me praising the Lord on the praise team. It was rough. The person that I had trusted more than anyone else, had betrayed that trust. The future that I had envisioned was suddenly nonexistent. I thought that we had a good marriage. Even though things had been rough lately, I figured if this was going on, he would want to work it out. I couldn't have been more wrong. He wanted out of the marriage. I was broken hearted. All of a sudden, I had no husband and no parents. I'll say here:

"When you're drowning in life's situations
just remember one thing....
your lifeguard walks on water."

I was up, off and on, all night. I kept praying for God to let me stop Mike from preaching. I felt I heard God say in my spirit, "No, I can use sinful man." I had wanted to get the DVD from the PI and when Mike asked to show the video from Burundi, the DVD of him and the other woman would come on the screen. I guess God didn't want that to happen. Personally, I wanted that. Oh well, I did pray for God's perfect will. I finally fell asleep.

Sunday morning, March 12, 2006, couldn't come soon enough. On the way to church I asked Mike if he was spiritually ready to be in the pulpit. He was taken aback.

He asked, "Why are you asking me that?" I told him, "I believe the pulpit at Crossroads is a very holy place and you are getting ready to step into it and preach." I sort of enjoyed watching him squirm. I guess I was hoping he would break down, confess, and say that he couldn't preach with this on his conscience. Instead, he did the usual and turned it back on me. He smirked and turned away. He acted like I was so mean to him. Again, he was angry at me. Funny, I was sitting there asking him about his spiritual condition and I'm mean.

Mike spoke in Sunday School. I remember looking at him as he stood in front of the Young Married class with disbelief. How could he be so calm and arrogant? He was having an adulterous affair yesterday, yet today was standing before this large class, acting like he was so holy. He was telling these young couples how to have a good marriage - definitely surreal. I don't remember what he said or what he taught on. My mind was racing.

This same morning he also preached in big church and showed the Burundi video. At the beginning of his sermon his dad was taking what Mike thought was too long to introduce him preaching, so Mike walked out onto the platform. He angrily grabbed the microphone from Dan saying, "You're preaching my sermon." Watching him standing up there in front of the entire church, I realized he was different. Then it dawned on me that maybe I'm different. Scripture tells us we see through the glass darkly. Well let me tell you when you see clearly through the glass – it is eye opening! Mike kept sweating and wiping his brow. Interesting. I prayed that as he gave his altar call, he would be humbled – but no.

We ate at Willow Creek with his family. We took our usual nap. I laid facing away from Mike with my eyes wide open. I now knew what all I had to do tomorrow. I had started my list, written in shorthand of course, so he couldn't read it. The evening service ended up with a lot of singing. I sang for an hour and a half, but finally I left because I truly felt sick. I'm sure from lack of sleep and stress. I told Terri and Steve on the phone. I was up all night thinking and praying. I didn't sleep. Terri and I kept texting. I have a list of things to do in the morning before I can confront him. Every minute gets harder. I know God is carrying me through this whirlwind of emotion and pain. I would be in a ball on the floor if Jesus weren't giving me wisdom, strength and peace. Thank you Lord.

Monday, March 13, 2006, as I took my bath, Mike sorted the laundry. "Appropriate," I thought. "He needs to learn to do his own laundry." I began putting on my makeup, but before Mike left for work, he came back into the bathroom. He walked over to where I was sitting at my makeup table. He grabbed my face with both hands, turned my face toward him, and said, "I *want* to be married to you." I answered sarcastically and sourly, "How sweet." It was all I could muster.

I took Sesily to Carl's Jr. for breakfast and then to her Driver's Ed class. I met the PI and saw his video on the tiny screen of his camera. She looks small, but I couldn't tell who she was and I didn't recognize the car. I went to the bank and got *all* our liquid cash so that I can stay in this house, purchased new doorknobs so the doors will lock, called the locksmith, and talked to an attorney named Arnold Fagan.

I told Duke over the phone. I think I wanted someone to know before I called Mike to come home, in case something went terribly wrong. I called Mike. Interestingly, he didn't even question why I was asking him to, but he came home and I confronted him. As I already said, I think he knew that I knew.

He wouldn't admit it for half an hour. At first I didn't tell him that I had proof. I wanted to see if he would come clean or just lie like he did when he was talking to the other woman.

For 25 minutes, he tried to deny it. He talked, but didn't tell me anything. I think he was trying to figure out what I knew. It seemed like he wanted to lie his way through it, but needed to know what I knew. Finally, when I said I had proof, he admitted it who it was with. He said that the affair has gone on for 8 months - since last July.

The lock guy called right as we were leaving to go talk to Dan and Bonnie. I think most men would have waited to go talk to their parents, but not Mike. He left. I was relieved. I had Doc pick up Sesily, and we all met here at the house about 1 PM. Mike returned and he told Sesily, Doc and Cami that he'd been having, "an adulterous affair." Duke came in a little later. He told Dan and Bon, or said he did. What do I do now? I'm numb.

Somehow through this ordeal of figuring out if he was being unfaithful, I kept a pretty good attitude and continued to laugh. After it was all out, I had some really rough moments here and there, but I think I knew the best way through this quagmire was to do what I have always done, and to just keep smiling... and hold my head high. My children and grandchildren would come over and we were able to laugh and cut-up. Don't get me wrong, we cried too, but we didn't stay in that place of pain. I knew that even though we didn't understand everything, God would work it for our good.

> *"And we know that in all things*
> *God works for the good of those*
> *who love him, who have been called*
> *according to his purpose."*
> *Romans 8:28*

God had His hand on us even when we didn't understand it.

Soon after Mike's parents rejected me too. They blamed me for everything. This was by far *the* most painful thing I'd experienced. His parents had become my parents. Bonnie wouldn't speak to me at church or at Praise Team practice. Bonnie, Dan, and I did try to talk a couple of times but we always ended up mad.

To this day, I'm still not sure exactly what Mike told them because I wasn't there. I think he let them know that he didn't want to work it out with me. One of the narcissistic comments he did say to me was that if he couldn't keep his job, then he didn't want to work it out.

That was the wrong thing to say to me. It let me know what I had known throughout our entire marriage of 30 years – that his job meant more to him than I did. If you believe actions speak louder than words, he had been showing me this for years. I kept trying to believe his words. A few months later I heard the quote but forgot to write down the author:

Don't believe
what someone says.
Believe what they do.

That has become my mantra. There is so much truth in that!

Do not be anxious about anything,
but in everything by
prayer and supplication
with thanksgiving
let your requests
be made known to God.
Phil. 4:6 ESV

It is hard to not be anxious when you are going through problems. Keep in mind, I knew how to get through difficulty. After everything I had already been through, I felt I could handle just about anything.

I know this is pretty heavy – the wondering, the waiting, the pain of the person you trust the most betraying you. I've told you some of the terrible things that have happened, but I definitely don't want to leave out the other side of that.

The Lord is close
to the ***brokenhearted***
and saves those
who are crushed in spirit.
Psalm 34:18 NIV

It was hard, however, God helped me and my family through it. He was close to us in our heartbreak. He was right there as we were crushed. I'm thankful I know Him and that we had Him to help us.

Whatever you are going through, God will be right beside you. He is there every step of the way. As I counsel people going through terrible situations, I urge them to look for the good. I advise them to look for what I call God winks - Squire Rushnell's term he explains like this:

An event or personal experience, often identified as coincidence, so astonishing that it is seen as a sign of divine intervention, especially when perceived as the answer to a prayer.

That's where something happens that means something to only you – like a message from God.

When you are in the middle of one of your life's darkest moments, a tiny message straight from God for you is one of the most comforting things I've ever experienced. It let me know that God had His eyes on me and he knew what I was going through. Yes, it was bleak and dark. I wasn't sure how it was all going to turn out, but knowing that God knew where I was and was sending me a message, was amazing!

Even in the darkness, it is best to…

keep smiling…

<u>Proverbs 6:32-33</u>

**Adultery is a brainless act,
soul-destroying, self-destructive;
Expect a bloody nose, a black eye,
and a reputation ruined for good. MSG**

Chapter 11 –
Maybe There's a Better Door

When my marriage ended, I thought my life was over. It became clear pretty rapidly that even though my husband claimed he would be going through the Assemblies of God restoration program and work on our marriage, he wasn't doing any of it. He simply got the information so he could show it to his parents and tell *them* he was going to. This all of a sudden seemed quite familiar – saying the right thing, but not doing the right thing. In those first few days he did invite me to his hotel room, but I just couldn't go. It was strange. I wanted to go, but knew it was best if I didn't. It was like the Lord prevented me from going. His paramour was like cocaine to him. He couldn't stop himself. I wanted him to fight for me and for our family and for our relationship. It never happened. Rejection is a soul wound. It hurts in the deepest parts of you.

I was sad but God was so good to me during this time. I'd like to also look back with 20/20 vision at the amazing and wonderful times where God was close to me and blessed me. Going through something this terrible changes your perspective. I'm sure it is the same if you discover you or your child has an incurable disease. In a Nano-second everything becomes crystal clear.

What came clear to me was to keep my family close and to lead them in such a way that they would be proud of me. My parents had passed away years before and I think somewhere in my mind, I also felt like they were watching. I wanted them to be proud of me too. The Message Bible says it like this,

> *Parents rejoice when their children turn out well; Wise children become proud parents. So make your father happy! Make your mother proud! Proverbs 23:23-25 MSG*

This dark period of my life taught me that the only one we can depend on is Jesus. Fortunately for me, I didn't have my eyes on my husband or his father, who was my pastor at the time this was happening. I had my eyes fully fixed on Jesus. I had met Jesus and asked him into my heart when I was 16. I truly met Him. He was my constant companion. That right there is reason enough to keep smiling and basically I did. I didn't know what the future held, but I knew Jesus would take care of me through whatever was coming.

As I laid in bed one evening, I felt like God was holding me in His arms. It was just what I needed. Mike wasn't there for me, but God was and I was grateful.

A few days later on Thursday, March 16, 2006, Mike met with Wayne & Nilo, two Deacon Board Members, and they asked him to resign. Mike acted to me like he was surprised they had ask him to resign. Duh. Seriously? When we were having this discussion, Mike asked me to dinner. I said no and then he cried. What?! Finally a tear from him. This was the first time he shed a tear, except when he told the kids and I felt that was simply shame not sorrow. These tears were still not for me, but for his job. He begged me to go to dinner. I finally said yes. When I did, he added, "I want to go, if you won't bludgeon me." He said he wanted to go "for some conversation." After he said all that, I said I wasn't sure I could do that, so no. He came over for more clothes. He was always trying to control the situation.

I struggled through these first few months because I had the desire to save my 35 year relationship. I am a person of action and I wanted to do something to save it. Every time I tried, it was met with cruelty and emotionless reactions from him. It was like Mike was blank and empty. He was uncaring and detached from me and the kids. As usual, he had absolutely nothing to give emotionally. This should have told me how things were going to turn out, but I clung to hope somehow, that with God's help, we could navigate these dicey waters.

Mike and I had tried to discuss things a few times beyond that first conversation. We eventually went to dinner about a week later for a "date." I had told him we needed to start from the beginning. It didn't end well. I had driven my own car and quickly left after we started fighting. Another time at my suggestion, we attended The Bridge Church in Mustang. We did ride together that night. As we stood on the back row during praise and worship, Mike tried to slip his hand down the back of my pants. I was horrified and turned to stop him. He thought it was hilarious! I thought it showed his disrespect for me. Here he was treating me however he wanted, with no regard for what I wanted. I had expressed the need to "start over" with our relationship and a new relationship didn't include things like that!!!

When we went to The Bridge together, we had a fight in the car heading home as we were talking about how the board members had treated him in their meeting. He got overly defensive which I thought was strange. All the information was out there, so why act like you're innocent? It was difficult. When I got home I thought to myself, "Don't ever get in the car with him again." I didn't want to be trapped like that. I didn't. It was this evening that made me realize we probably would never be able to work the relationship out – not that I wasn't willing. It was more about how we saw things so differently and his need to control. He did not care about the covenant we had made. He did not care about the pain he was inflicting on me and his family.

After our Ted's date, when I left, I went to Doc and Cami's for pizza. Trip, my first grandson, was so funny. He kept me laughing even in the midst of all my pain. Thank you God for my family. They are such a joy and comfort to me. I kept praying for God to help me through this. My prayer seems to continually end with, "Lord, I can't go through this again, so if he is ever going to be unfaithful to me again, I want to cut my losses now." I am sure part of that comes from the fact that he had done this to me before in 1989 with the other woman

When someone is going through a personal battle like this, God obviously has faith in you as a warrior. He knows you will be taking some serious blows. He also knows you can take it! You must keep your faith alive and well. There will be dark days. There will be moments you are not sure you're going to make it!

Keep your head up.

Ask God for guidance, strength, direction, and perseverance.

Some battles require tenacity. That is the ability to stick with something. Every day something would happen to break my heart once more. However, every morning the sun came up and it was a good day. There was laughter and joy. Trip was about 13 months old when this happened. He was so wonderful at taking all my thoughts and putting them totally on him! He would giggle and my broken heart would burst with joy. It's funny how that works. You can be brokenhearted and joyful all at once!

One day soon after he had learned to walk Trip was trying to get to my telephone which I kept on the marble behind the tub. It was raised about 18 inches. He eyed it for a bit, then got to work. He got on his hands and knees and pushed my scales over toward the bath. The scales were probably 4 inches tall. He stepped on them and to his delight, he could now reach the telephone. Jubilation was written on that sweet innocent face! I loved that his little analytical mind was already working to solve problems.

It let me know that our minds are powerful. I was overwhelmed when I considered all my current problems, but I knew that my powerful mind would help me figure all this out. I knew God would let me know what I needed to do at the right time. It gave me peace. A serenity of knowing God was in charge and He would take care of all the details.

My children surrounded me with love in a way that I never imagined. The 6 of us grew closer than ever before. I think we needed each other. We knew that life as we had known it was over. We were unsure of what lay ahead. It was frightening and we needed one another. My friends became more than friends. They were a lifeline that truly kept me afloat.

It reminded me of the story of the four friends who wanted their friend to be healed. He couldn't get to

Jesus on his own, so they carried him and brought their friend to Jesus to be healed from Mark 2 or Luke 5. The problem was the door was blocked.

> *Since they could not get him to Jesus because of the crowd, they made an opening in the roof above Jesus by digging through it and then lowered the mat the man was lying on.*
> *Mark 2:4 NIV*

> *When they could not find a way to do this because of the crowd, they went up on the roof and lowered him through the tiles into the middle of the crowd, right in front of Jesus. Luke 5:19*

Instead of taking their friend back home and giving up, these friends went up on the roof and made a way. They forced it. They didn't abandon their friend.

They loved their friend too much to turn away and miss the opportunity for him to be healed. Most of us know the rest of the story. One unusual part of it is in verse 5 where it says,

> *"When Jesus saw their faith..." [Their meaning the friends' faith,] "He said to the paralyzed man, 'Son, your sins are forgiven.'"*

I find it interesting because the friends had a big part to play. It was "*their*" faith, the friends' faith, that moved Jesus. Don't think you are not doing enough when you are just there with your friend who is suffering! Because of their friends' determination and love, the man got up, took his mat and walked out of the very doorway that had previously blocked him!!!

At this time in my life, I felt paralyzed - much like that man. However, with my friends near, I knew I could walk through this door and if I couldn't walk, they would carry me. Where would this new door lead? What did the future hold? Which way should I go? I wasn't sure what lay ahead, but I knew I would be okay!

My family and my friends carried me through some of my life's darkest moments. I'm so thankful they were there. During this period I learned that with family and friends there, you can always

keep smiling…

Be strong and of good courage;
do not be afraid, nor be dismayed,
for the Lord your God
is with you wherever you go.
Joshua 1:9

Chapter 12
A Bad Situation

I knew how to get through difficulty. After my grandmother and dad died within a week and a few years later my mother and her mom died the same day, and my second child telling me he's gay, I felt like I could handle just about anything. I knew whatever came my way wasn't fatal. I also believed that God can repair any relationship. I was broken- hearted, and I was not in any way able to repair it myself. I was waiting for my husband to step up and fight for our 35 years together. He never did.

It was during these first few weeks after discovering the affair that I began to listen not only to what God was saying to me, but I was listening to myself. What was *I* saying about Sandy? The powerful voice inside your head is usually the one you end up listening to. I found I had been agreeing with Mike. I was telling myself I wasn't good enough, I wasn't skinny enough, or I wasn't worth fighting for. I had to make a concentrated effort to stop saying such negative things. I caught the end of a program on letting God talk to you. He explained that most of the time this would happen about 3 A.M., because that's when we're available.

I began waking up at about that time. I would get my support pillow and actually sit up in bed. I knew if I didn't, I would fall back asleep. In the darkness I would listen to what God had to say to me. He never told me *I* wasn't good enough or skinny enough or wasn't worth fighting for. He was reminding me that *I* was fearfully and wonderfully made.

> *I praise you because I am fearfully and wonderfully made; your works are wonderful, I know that full well. Psalm 139:14 NIV*

God would remind me that all of this mess would work together for my good.

> *And we know that all things work together for good to those who love God, to those who are the called according to his purpose.*
> *Romans 8:28-29 NIV*

He would jog my memory to not be afraid.

> *Be strong and of good courage; do not be afraid, not be dismayed, for the Lord your God is with you wherever you go. Joshua 1:9*

These middle of the night "talks" with the Lord became my lifeline. I would look forward to them. I would find myself wondering what else He would have to say.

I should point out here that in our middle of the night talks, the Lord always had something positive to say to me, as you can tell from the scriptures above. They were always uplifting. God would give me fantastic ideas and when I woke up, I would somehow believe that I could do them. These talks were so needed. The previous two years with my husband giving me very little time or attention and rarely showing me authentic appreciation, had squashed my self-esteem down to nothing! Self-esteem is your opinion of yourself. My ex had convinced me that I was worthless. Feeling insignificant was wearing on the quality of my life.

I had always thought highly of myself. In junior high and high school I was a cheerleader who loved to lead the crowds in cheers. I enjoyed smiling and trying to pep up the people who had come to the games. After I got married I felt pretty important as a wife and mother and as a pastor's wife. I played the piano and sang for the church. I felt the calling on my life was purposeful. Throughout the 30 years of marriage, but especially in the past two years, I became convinced that I was of little value. Now I know that most mothers go through this as the nest becomes empty. I still had one child at home, but she was a teenager and didn't need me as much. I began to feel this way and didn't know what to do about it.

I was searching for answers from my husband, but he sadly, had nothing to give me. I had always said his parents were emotionally unavailable, but I was now realizing that he was too. It was too much. I needed him and he simply wasn't there for me. I would try to explain what I needed, but it was as if he couldn't hear me. Maybe he didn't want to hear me. How can you give something you don't have? You can't. He wasn't able to give me what he didn't have in him.

When I look back now, I can see that we both desperately needed something from one another, yet we didn't know how to give what the other needed. How strangely sad. How extraordinarily tragic. Our once fabulous relationship was crumbling and neither one of us knew how to stop it. I was not okay and neither was he.

Here's a poem I wrote of my despair:

FOG

I look out my window and see fog.
Nothing else. Just fog.
No purpose – no plans – no nothing – just fog.
When did this fog set in?
Does it matter? I'm in it.
It engulfs me, strangling the very life from my being.
I go through motions.
Smiles, words, movements
but there is no life – just fog.
Empty, I stare at the people watching me
wondering why no one recognizes the emptiness.
Maybe they don't want to see it.
Maybe they do see
and just don't know what to do.
The word zombie is appropriate here.
One who moves as if alive
but really isn't;
a mechanical man; one on automation.
Definitely me.
Fog woman – that's me.
Some say "be happy."
Okay. Gee, why didn't I think of that?
I do try, but when I try
there is no life to sustain its drive.
Only more fog.
I wait patiently for the sun to come again.
God make it come quickly because I'm dying here.

He claimed at our only counseling session that it began when my mother died. Maybe he was right. She used to fill my love tank. Now there was no one to fill it. Mike was emotionally unavailable and wasn't able to.

I was looking for the woman I had previously been, but she was not there. I had always enjoyed volunteering and entertaining, but now I no longer wanted to do these things. This was a challenge I was unaccustomed to. I even told Mike that he had finally won me over to being just like him, meaning that I didn't want to socialize. My enthusiasm for life was gone.

It took heavenly conversations to rebuild the personality parts that had been destroyed. I had been wounded to my very core. It took TBN and Daystar being on my television all the time. I only listened to uplifting music. I was listening to the Lord tell me who I was instead of listening to that cruel and negative voice of some people around me. God was telling me who I was, instead of a man. I got reacquainted with who I truly was on the inside. It was needed. I slowly began to remember this person inside of me and I liked her! The circumstances that had knocked me down did not have control over my core person. I had control of that!

This was great news because frankly at this point in my life, I didn't have control over much. My ex-husband had put me in a situation that was scary. When I was put onto that roller coaster ride, I had to make a decision and I had to maintain the right attitude when the going got rough. I decided early-on through that terribly negative situation that the ***only*** thing I could control was my attitude. So I began to control that.

My family was my saving grace. They would come over or we would go out to eat, and we would laugh it up. We would even crack jokes about our horrible circumstances. The great thing was that we could laugh about it. We were all able to **keep smiling.** This was miraculous!

I honestly believe God allowed us to see the humor in it. I mean, think about it. Here is a God fearing Assembly of God family whose father and husband, a well-respected pastor, has had an affair and is now going off on his own to start a new life without all of us! I'm pretty sure God was shaking his head in disbelief. This man had portrayed Jesus! I used to enjoy telling people that I slept with Jesus! Lol It always got a good laugh. This was the man teaching our young couples how to have a good marriage. It really was humorous! I'm sure the devil was really laughing!

This was the time in my life that I realized I had to take control over my thoughts, so I did. L

> *Casting down imaginations and every high thing that exalteth itself against the knowledge of God, and bringing into captivity every thought to the obedience of Christ... 2 Cor. 10:5 KJV*

Perhaps you need to take back control over your thoughts. Your opinion of yourself is of utmost importance. Sometimes we allow other people's opinions to be the most dominant. Don't get me wrong, it is nice when men speak well of you. However, scripture says to be careful of that!

> *Woe to you when all men speak well of you, For so did their fathers to the false prophets.*
> *Luke 6:26*

I think the Message Bible says it best,

> *There's trouble ahead when you live only for the approval of others, saying what flatters them, doing what indulges them. Popularity contests are not truth contests—look how many scoundrel*

preachers were approved by your ancestors! Your task is to be true, not popular. Luke 6:26 MSG

Don't worry about what others think of you. Only be concerned with what God thinks of you. When you do this, all other relationships come in line with what is most important.

Another issue I struggled with was forgiveness. I knew I was commanded to forgive. Matthew 5:44-48 tells us to:

Love your enemies, bless them that curse you,
do good to them that hate you,
and pray for them which despitefully use you,
and persecute you;
That ye may be the children of your Father
which is in heaven: for he maketh his sun to rise
on the evil and on the good,
and sendeth rain on the just and on the unjust.
For if ye love them which love you,
what reward have ye?
do not even the publicans the same?
And if ye salute your brethren only, what do ye
more than others? do not even the publicans so?
Be ye therefore perfect,
even as your Father which is in heaven is perfect.
Matthew 5:44-48

I had to work at it. It didn't come naturally for me. As usual, I turned to the scriptures. 1 Cor. 13:5 in each of the following bibles spoke right to the heart of my wounded soul. 1 Cor. 13:5 in the ASV says,

..doth not behave itself unseemly
(unbecoming), seeketh not its own,
is not provoked, taketh not account of evil;..
I Cor. 13:5 ASV

The Message bible explains it like this:

Doesn't keep score of the sins of others,
Doesn't revel when others grovel...
I Cor. 13:5 MSG

Here is the Amplified version:

...it does not take into account a wrong endured... I Cor. 13:5 AMP

Kenneth Hagin's book <u>Love the Way to Victory</u> says,

"This is the divine love gauge."

Our human instincts are the opposite. We want to keep score. We look for the worst in others and the best in ourselves. Some look at this as weakness. We say things like, "He's a pushover..." or "She's a doormat.." We must recognize that God doesn't remember their wrongs, so why should we? If you do, *you* are not walking in love.

I know exactly what you're thinking because I thought it too. Why should I forgive someone who has wronged me on such a horrendous level? I generally explain that my husband's affair was a pain that wounded me to the very core of who I was. It was an injury so deep and so hurtful, I truly wondered if I would ever recover. This was the man that I had trusted with my deepest darkest feelings and fears. This was the person on the planet that I *thought* I could rely on. When he betrayed me, it was an injury that although there was no outer wound, there was deep internal bleeding that I wasn't sure at the time could be healed. So trying to forgive him seemed impossible. How do you not keep score of a wound like that? How do I forgive him?

This goes against our human nature. We want God to remember that wrong. This part was tough for me. If you have been mistreated and I mean really wronged, this is extremely difficult. Please understand me here, I have learned to forgive. I have learned to pray for those like it tells us to in Matthew 5:44:

But I say to you, love your enemies,
bless those who curse you,
do good to those who hate you,
and pray for those who spitefully
use you and persecute you... Matthew 5:44

I've got this one down. I've also tried doing what James 1:2-4 says,

Consider it nothing but joy, my brothers and sisters, whenever you fall into various trials. Be assured that the testing of your faith [through experience] produces endurance [leading to spiritual maturity, and inner peace]. And let endurance have its perfect result and do a thorough work, so that you may be perfect and completely developed [in your faith] lacking in nothing. James 1:2-4 AMP

I have tried to live Romans 12:19,

Beloved, do not avenge yourselves, but rather
give place to wrath; for it is written,
"Vengeance is Mine, I will repay,"
Romans 12:19

See all of these scriptures fit perfectly into my way of thinking, that what someone did to me was bad, and they should be punished!

Brother Hagin said on page 10 of this book:

> *"As long as you're taking into account of the evil done to you, you're not walking in love... As long as you're taking account of the evil done to you, you won't be able to believe the best of every person... God's love is ever ready to believe the best about every person. Since God is love, that means God is ever ready to believe the best about each one of us."*

Talk about a two-edged sword. I want God to love me and think the best of me. Yet in that same breath, I find myself thinking I'm better than someone else because I didn't do what that they did. But this book reminded me that God loves them just as much as He loves me.

If someone mistreats a member of my family, things are not going to be good between me and that person. They're just not! If someone mistreats a member of your family –then things are not good between you and that person, right? That's how God looks at it. If you mistreat someone God loves, He is not okay with you!!! We are all God's children. If His children are mistreated, He's not okay with it – even if they've wronged you. Even if they're not living for the Lord. Even if they're outright sinners.

By ***this*** *we know that we know Him, if we keep His commandments. He who says, "I know Him," and does not keep His commandments, is a liar, and the truth is not in him. But whoever keeps His word, truly the love of God is perfected in him. By this we know that we are in Him. 6 He who says he abides in Him ought* *himself also to walk just as He walked. Brethren, I write* ***no new commandment*** *to you, but* ***an old commandment which you have had from the beginning****. (The beginning of Jesus' ministry). The old commandment is the word which you heard from the beginning. Again, a new commandment I write to you, which thing is true in Him and in you, because the darkness is passing away, and the true light is already shining. He who says he is in the light, and hates his brother, is in darkness until now. He who loves his brother abides in the light, and there is no cause for stumbling in him. But he who hates his brother is in darkness and walks in darkness, and does not know where he is going, because the darkness has blinded his eyes.   I John 2:3-9 NKJV*

This puts it in a whole new perspective. We are to LOVE them all!!! Love them with an unconditional love! For God so loved... I want to add: only those who are living right... only those who are doing right? No! For God so loved the world!!! That He gave His only begotten son, that whosoever... That whosoever includes the person that has wronged you. That can be hard to swallow, but it's true.

We are all God's children. As humans we understand that if one of our kids messes up, it never removes our love for them. When I came to grips with this, I knew that I had to forgive. I wanted forgiveness for all *my* wrongs – the ones I have done in my life. I had to forgive my ex to be able to move forward with my life, and to be in a place to receive what God had for me. I had to learn to love them.

At first I would pray for them and they were just words with very little meaning. However, the more I prayed, the easier it became. It didn't happen overnight.

It takes time. There's that word again – time. I heard someone say to:

Give time - time.

It's true because at some point, I actually meant the prayers. I could truly wish them well. I could do this. I could forgive. I could leave all of my pain and anger at Jesus' feet. I could hand over my desire for vengeance to a good and just God.

Once I did that, I started healing in a new and different way. God was helping me. I had to walk in love. I John 2:3-9 says it like this:

> *If you will forgive, you will be able to move forward. Even if you never speak to that person and tell them what you have done. This is for you and you alone, not for them. Begin to love as Christ loves. It will make a difference.*
> *I John 2:3-9*

If you are not there yet, give yourself some grace. My ability to forgive ebbs and flows, even to this day many years later. I have days that unforgiveness rears its ugly head. I have other days that I am strong and sure of the forgiveness I have offered. God looks on the heart. He understands where you are and how you are feeling and coping with your situations. Wherever you are on your journey to healing and wholeness, know that God will meet you on that road. He never sleeps and will be there whenever you need Him.

I'm so thankful that God was right there to help me rediscover who I really am. He will do the same for you, but you must be willing forgive and to listen. He will be there for you to, but we must make time for Him. We must create a space where there are no distractions.

No phone calls, no television, no diversions. Just you and the Lord. Alone. With you praying… And mainly listening for His divine guidance.

Now it's your turn. Close this book and turn everything off. "Wait" upon the Lord. Stay in a place of expectation. Ready for a word from Him. Remember He will never give you anything to go against what He has already written. Prepare for what He is going to tell you. It can be several nights before you hear anything, but continue to read His word and then wait… and while you're waiting for Him, remember to…

keep smiling…

It's funny but as I lay here in the dark,
I have peace –
the kind that passes all understanding.
It is real rest in God.
I know that even though
I don't understand one thing
happening to me,
God is guiding me.
I'm lost in certain ways because I don't know
where I am or where I'm going.
Yet, I know that God knows.
I wake up every day and say, "Lead on!"

Chapter 13 – "Lead On Lord..."

Here is an excerpt from my journal:

One of the wise older church ladies called and prophesied over me. She said I'm like Esther. That I have been called for such a time as this.

> *...And who knows but that you have come to your royal position for such a time as this?*
> *Esther 4:4 NIV*

That scripture is certainly my prayer. All I could do was cry as she talked to me. If she is right perhaps someday all of this will make sense. This situation was actually another opportunity to believe God has only good things in store for me. In the story of David and Goliath, David could have cowered in fear with the rest of the soldiers, but he chose to believe God was who He said He was!!! The two thieves that were on the cross with Jesus had the opportunity to choose. One chose to believe and the other chose not to.

Here is what I wrote in my diary on May 20, 2006, when I was in the middle of all this:

*May 20, 2006 Saturday I woke up @ 5 AM and read the Bible. I got flowers to plant after I worked on my Sunday School lesson. We shopped at Penn Square after we lunch at Java Dave's. We saw Mike's car at an apartment complex near 89th & I-44. Bon called this morning and asked me "not to file for divorce." She wants me to "try and work it out." Unreal. This is the 1st conversation with her about fixing our relationship and it's 2 months in. I went to Ses' recital. Sesily's boyfriend Josh, Caleb, Rachel, Travis and I came. Josh brought flowers. Ses was going to invite Mike if he called her, but he never did. She didn't invite him to her Awards Ceremony either. We went to Hideaway Pizza with the Ferguson's and their friends Steve & Tammy. Fun! Sesily washed her hair. We went to bed at 11:30 PM.

It's funny but as I lay there in the dark, I have peace. The kind that passes all understanding. It is real rest in God. I know that even though I don't understand one thing that is happening to me, God is guiding me. I'm lost in certain ways because I don't know where I am or where I'm going. Yet, I know that God knows. I wake up every day and say, **"Lead on!"**

I truly, for the first time in my life, know that I have my hand in the hand of the one who calmed the waters. It is so comforting. I am sad because things are not happening the way I want and yet in that sadness, there is peace that everything is happening exactly the way God wants it to. Weird? Yes! Wonderful? Yes! Comforting? Absolutely! Lead On…*

Notice how in the middle of terrible circumstances and pain, we were still enjoying life. I had tried to make that a priority with my family! We were going to spend time with friends and we were trying to keep busy. I refused to sit in my rocking chair and cry. I kept living and enjoying life! Certain incidents had occurred which were extremely painful to walk through. I was reading

Streams in the Desert by L.B. Cowman and Forgive and Forget by Lewis Smedes. People had given me books that had helped them through tough times and I was reading every word!

I love this from *Streams in the Desert*:

"Through the leaves of every trial there are chinks of light to shine through. Thorns do not prick you unless you lean against them, and not one touches without His knowledge. The words that hurt you, the letter which gave you pain, the cruel wound of your dearest friend, shortness of money–are all known to Him, who sympathizes as no one else can and watches to see, if, through all, you will dare to trust Him wholly."

Could I dare to trust Him? I determined to. Lewis B. Smedes offers this quote from *Forgive and Forget*:

"Forgiving is love's toughest work, and love's biggest risk. If you twist it into something it was never meant to be, it can make you a doormat or an insufferable manipulator. Forgiving seems almost unnatural. Our sense of fairness tells us people should pay for the wrong they do. But forgiving is love's power to break nature's rule."

This turned out to be very true. Forgiving *is* love's toughest work. I would find myself wishing that I had the opportunity to forgive Mike. Then at the same moment worry whether I could actually do it. I didn't know. We are commanded to forgive, but what he had done hurt worse than any pain I had suffered in my life. I definitely needed God's help in this.

During this time I remembered years ago reading books by Barbara Johnson. Several of her quotes which follow would bring me a giggle at certain times:

"Remember to keep the main thing the main thing.

Laughter is to life what shock absorbers are to automobiles. It won't take the potholes out of the road, but it sure makes the ride smoother.

Whatever it is probably won't go away, so we might as well live and laugh through it. When we double over laughing, we're bending so we won't break. If you think your particular troubles are too heavy and too traumatic to laugh about, remember that laughing is like changing a baby's diaper. It doesn't solve any problems permanently, but it makes things more acceptable for a while.

Faith is seeing light with your heart when all your eyes see is darkness.

It never hurts your eyesight to look on the bright side of things.

We cannot protect ourselves from trouble, but we can dance through the puddles of life with a rainbow smile, twirling the only umbrella we need -- the umbrella of God's love."

I was so glad I had read her books when all this was revealed. I had read some previously, but they were now a healing balm to my wounded soul. Only eternity will reveal the people she helped through hard times. She had many hard times in her life too, yet she was determined to only look on the bright side! I resolved to do the same. I was closer to God than I ever had been in my life. I prayed daily for God's help and guidance.

Approximately a year later in May of 2007 I also wrote in my journals: *Cami and Doc went for an ultrasound today and found out Shaylee has a lot of fuzz (hair)! So exciting! Trip, now 2, knows his whole alphabet except he says horse for H, Zebra for Z and Monkey for M. He is a genius! Doc passed his fireman's written test – yea! There were 400 who took the test and only 100 went on. He's prepping for the physical test on Saturday and has hurt his foot and tailbone – poor baby! Marcia Aycock and I are considering turning in papers for licenses with the Assemblies of God.*

See, in the middle of all this craziness, there's a great deal of positive things happening too! I always want to think on the good!

Sometimes we are so busy worrying about where we want to be or where we used to be that we forget being in the moment. Enjoy this moment no matter what you are going through and…

keep smiling…

"I don't know what has broken your heart or what loss has come to you, but I do know that God wants to come to the tomb of that loss in this season of your life, minister His own presence to you there and bring a delivery out of that tomb…"

- Beth Moore

Chapter 14 –
The Stone is Rolled Back

Easter. What an amazing time of year, especially for the Christian. Jesus had lived 33 years and had an amazing 3 year ministry. Things were going great for Jesus. Remember the triumphant entry into Jerusalem? His disciples probably had no clue things were going to go south quickly!

The next day the huge crowd that had arrived for the Feast heard that Jesus was entering Jerusalem. They broke off palm branches and went out to meet him. And they cheered:

> *Hosanna!*
> *Blessed is he who comes in God's name!*
> *Yes! The King of Israel!*
> *John 12:12-13 MSG*

Jesus was on top of the world... For a moment in time... Within the week he was arrested and beaten almost to death. He was offered to be released to this same crowd, but the mob chose Barabbas! The very same crowd who had loved him, and shouted adoring phrases and offered palm branches, now wanted him dead. Jesus was crucified a few days later. I'm sure to some, all hope was lost when Jesus said, *"It is finished."*

Let's face it, people are fickle. My husband was fickle. Just as Jesus had experienced this, so had I.

Easter had never been more real to me. The suffering, the people changing their mind, the betrayal – it was very real.

Isaiah 53 says that Jesus was a man of sorrows and acquainted with grief. Many Christ followers say, "I want to be like Jesus" or "I want to be more like Jesus. We wear bracelets that ask the question, "What Would Jesus Do?" Maybe you remember the old worship song that goes:

I wanna be more like You, Jesus
I wanna be more like You, Jesus
I wanna be a vessel You work through,
I wanna be more like You.

Do we really? Are we serious?

Because Jesus had to go through a lot of bad stuff. Jesus had to ride a roller coaster. He entered Jerusalem with a palm branch parade and one week later that same crowd was shouting for his death and crucifixion.

Talk about a roller coaster. He could have been elected Mayor one day and within the week, the crowd wanted to kill him and beat him and put him on a cross. Isaiah 53:7 says "He was oppressed and He was afflicted, Yet He opened not His mouth…"

It's great to talk about being like Jesus when we picture Him sitting beside the right hand of God… Or when we want blessings and honor and glory. Bring it on, we want to be like Jesus - the resurrected Lord that gets the standing ovation at the end of every Easter Pageant - *that* is the Jesus we want to be like.
Not *this* one in Isaiah 53:3-12 NKJV:

He is despised and rejected by men,
A man of sorrows and acquainted with grief.
And we hid, as it were, our faces from Him;
He was despised, and we did not esteem Him.
Surely He has borne our griefs and carried our sorrows;
Yet we esteemed Him stricken,
smitten by God and afflicted.
But He was wounded for our transgressions,
He was bruised for our iniquities;
The chastisement for our peace was upon Him,
And by His stripes we are healed.
All we like sheep have gone astray;
We have turned every one, to his own way;
And the Lord has laid on Him the iniquity of us all.
He was oppressed and he was afflicted,
Yet He opened not His mouth,
He was led as a lamb to the slaughter,
and as a sheep before its shearers is silent,
so He opened not His mouth.
He was taken from prison and from judgment,
and who will declare his generation?
For He was cut off from the land of the living;
For the transgressions of My people He was stricken.
And they made His grave with the wicked –
But with the rich at His death,
Because He had done no violence,
nor was any deceit in His mouth.
Yet it pleased the Lord to bruise Him;
He has put Him to grief,
When You make His soul an offering for sin,
He shall see His seed,
He shall prolong His days, and the pleasure of the Lord shall prosper in His hand.
He shall see the travail of His soul and be satisfied.
By His knowledge My righteous Servant shall justify many, For He shall bear their iniquities.
Therefore I will divide Him a portion with the great,
And He shall divide the spoil with the strong.

Because He poured out His soul unto death,
And He was numbered with the transgressors,
And He bore the sin of many.
And made intercession for the transgressors.
Isaiah 53:3-12 NJKV

Now I don't know about you, but that is rough. We say we want to be like Jesus. Our prayer is often, "Lord make me more like you!" But this guy we just read about, this Jesus is bruised and broken, betrayed, and bloodied. He is scary. When I sing that song, "I wanna be more like You, Jesus" I'm talking about the good stuff, aren't you? This is a man who is despised – people can't stand him – I'm not sure I want to be like *Him*. They hate him. He is rejected of men. Most of us long for and want acceptance. We don't want to be rejected by our peers. Jesus was rejected. *This* is a man of sorrows.

Merriam Webster's dictionary says 'sorrow' means, "Mental pain, sadness, anguish and disappointment." He is acquainted with grief. That means Jesus is familiar with suffering, distress and heartache. He understands this on an even deeper level than what you are going through. He was sweating blood. When is the last time you were so upset, you were sweating blood? Read on. It says, we hid our faces from Him and did not esteem him. Have any of you ever felt like people were avoiding you? You looked at them, but they looked away and acted like they didn't see you. Most of us either as children or as adults have experienced that, and it is not pleasant. When it says they did not esteem him, that means they didn't appreciate him or give him any respect. He meant nothing to them. Baby that's low.

I felt pretty much like that from my in-laws and my husband. They previously loved me, but now - not so much! It was true betrayal. They wanted nothing to do with me. My mother-in-law wouldn't speak to me during Praise and Worship Team practice. We were at church when this was happening. My mother-in-law was older and knew better. I kept expecting more from her and was sorely disappointed. It was unreal. I felt I was getting the blame for something my husband had done. The pain was excruciating. I didn't know how to handle this kind of thing. I just had to breathe another breath and take another step. I just kept going. I was never rude to her. I just ignored her, like she was ignoring me. To me, it was heartbreaking. Looking back, I wish I had been the bigger person and treated her with love. I was too hurt to do that at this time.

Easter, is a reminder of the agonizing pain and betrayal that Jesus went through. Fortunately for us, however, the story doesn't end with pain and betrayal. Easter is not only about pain. Easter is about rebirth, resurrection, and restoration.

I want to repeat the quote that I gave at the beginning of this chapter, because it ministers to me so very much. Beth Moore was relating to Easter and everything Jesus had to go through. He was betrayed by those closest to him. I know it must have broken his heart. Those who had laid palm branches down for him to walk over just a few days before, were now yelling for his crucifixion. Even in the midst of this terrible ordeal, God sees what is on the other side. He will allow us to walk through painful places.

Beth Moore's quote says to let *Him* bring you back to life:

> *"I don't know what has broken your heart or what loss has come to you, but I do know that God wants to come to the tomb of that loss in this*

season of your life, minister His own presence to you there, and bring a delivery out of that tomb. God can bring new life to you and deliver you from this grief or this death. He IS the God of resurrection. Let Him bring you back to life!" - Beth Moore

Don't look at your circumstance as the end of your story. Look at it as the part right before your resurrection. Certainly, you may feel like giving up. You may feel boxed in and left for dead. It is often the time where you want to give up!

When you are going through this portion, and get impatient, remember God turns coal into diamonds, sand into pearls, and caterpillars into butterflies. All it takes is pressure and time.

If you're in the middle of something terrible, there's pressure. So all you and God need now - is time.

If you are like me, time passes *very* slowly when there is pain involved. Also unfortunately, patience is not one of my virtues. Just ask my family. In fact the whole Sheaffer family is not patient. I am, for sure, not patient at all. I want what I want and I want it now! I don't like waiting. I don't like waiting at the doctor's office, in the grocery store line, or even at a red light that takes too long. I consider this the worst part of whatever it is God is doing in me. Steven Furtick calls this painful time of pressure, "the dirt" as I said in Chapter 1. He says, "Let the dirt do its work. This is only a season for God to work in you and allow you to grow!"

As I mentioned before, waiting can be difficult. Patience is definitely a virtue and it's one that I do not possess. When I looked it up the word 'wait' means,

"Staying in a place of expectation. It means to be ready and available."

I don't know about you, but I think of waiting as a drudgery, and was surprised to see this definition. Staying in a place of expectation... that's great – if you're expecting something wonderful – like a new baby. However, what about while you're in prison... when you're in the pit... what are you expecting then? ... What about while things aren't happening like you thought they would. Joseph thought surely the baker or the cupbearer would remember to get him out of prison – especially since he had told them what their dreams meant and he was right. Yet it didn't turn out that way.

Let's face it, life oftentimes doesn't turn out like we think it is going to. It's so easy to say you trust Jesus. It is especially easy in the good times. However, when things aren't going well, it gets really hard. As believers, we should be able to trust Jesus in the good times AND in the hard times. It shouldn't matter what we're going through. When times are difficult, we complain and just want to get it over with. During these times, I don't ever feel like I'm in a place of hope and probability, waiting for something wonderful to come out of it.

Are you staying in a place of expectation? Are you ready and available for God to use you? Or are you like me and thinking of waiting as a drudgery? This verse actually says that those who wait receive fresh strength. Who wouldn't want that? When I looked up fresh, it means energetic, vigorous, lively. Strength means the state of being strong; having the power to resist attack; potency, might and vigor.

Yes, please, I would like all of the above, so help me Jesus to wait. This is where I really need God's assistance. I know I'm supposed to be in that place of expectation, but my lack of patience and my desire to get what I want right now, makes it hard to wait. I know I can do it with God's help! I certainly don't like a cake that hasn't been thoroughly cooked, but I do like brownies that are little under-done! Lol Okay, okay, I know you know what I mean!

Scripture says those who wait will spread their wings and soar like eagles. I think eagles are the most majestic bird out there. Did you know the eagle can fly carrying the heaviest load of any bird? Did you know eagles have eyes that can see twice as far as a human? Think of that, the eagle sees what other birds can't. Like us, as Christ followers, we should see a terrible situation and know that somehow - God is working in it.

Isaiah 40:29-31 in the Message Bible says it this way:

Don't you know anything?
Haven't you been listening?
God doesn't come and go. God lasts.
He's Creator of all you can see or imagine.
He doesn't get tired out,
doesn't pause to catch his breath.
And he knows everything, inside and out.
He energizes those who get tired,
gives fresh strength to dropouts.
For even young people tire and drop out,
young folk in their prime stumble and fall.
But those who wait upon God
get fresh strength.
They spread their wings
and soar like eagles.
They run and don't get tired,
they walk and don't lag behind.
Isaiah 40:29-31 MSG

Even if your situation is one that feels like the end. Perhaps you feel like you are boxed in and left for dead. Just remember Easter. It's not over. God will revive you, your faith, and your situation. We should keep in mind that the stone has been rolled away! It's done! He can restore whatever was broken. God will resurrect you in your situation and you *will* walk out of that tomb!

God has something wonderful in store for you, so all you need to do is wait and all you need to do in the waiting is to...

keep smiling...

Thou shalt love thy neighbor as thyself.
There is none other commandment
greater than these.
Mark 12:31 KJV

Chapter 15 – Love thy neighbor

Have you ever wondered why God put this verse in the Bible? I mean, think about it. We are to love God with all our heart, and with all thy soul, and with all thy might, is found in Deuteronomy 6:5 KJV That part is pretty easy! Then we're told to love our neighbor. That can be tough.

> *Love does no harm to a neighbor;*
> *Therefore love is the fulfillment of the law.*
> *Romans 13:10 NKJV*

People can be easy to love unless you live near them. I believe the scriptures teach us to love other people just as well as you do yourself. This is what we're *supposed* to do. The Message Bible explains it this way:

> *You can't go wrong when you love others.*
> *When you add up everything in the law code,*
> *the sum total is love. Romans 13:10 MSG*

I am fine when I'm reading about it. It sounds easy. Doing it is much harder than talking about it or reading scriptures about it.

The amplified version of the Bible continues this teaching:

"Owe nothing to anyone except to love and seek the best for one another; for he who [unselfishly] loves his neighbor has fulfilled the [essence of the] law [relating to one's fellowman]." The commandments, "You shall not commit adultery, you shall not murder, you shall not steal, you shall not covet," and any other commandment are summed up in this statement: "You shall love your neighbor as yourself." Love does no wrong to a neighbor [it never hurts anyone]. Therefore [unselfish] love is the fulfillment of the Law.
Romans 8:28-29 AMP

The KJV version says it like this,

"Owe no man anything, save to love one another: for he that loveth [d] his neighbor hath fulfilled the law. 9 For this, [e] Thou shalt not commit adultery, Thou shalt not kill, Thou shalt not steal, Thou shalt not covet, and if there be any other commandment, it is summed up in this word, namely, Thou shalt love thy neighbor as thyself. 10 Love worketh no ill to his neighbor: love therefore is the fulfilment of the law."
Romans 8:28-29 KJV

I always say that God ***had*** to put it in the bible to love your neighbor because it can be SO hard. I've known people who have put their house up for sale, because they couldn't get along with their neighbor. Let's face it, some neighbors - not you and me, of course - are hard to love!

My son, Duke, had a cursing verbal altercation with his neighbor over some bushes being trimmed and branches being dropped into his yard.

Another friend had issues with his neighbor playing loud music late into the night. Apparently the speaker was pointed directly at my friend's house.

Another friend had problems with their dog getting out, and the neighbor calling animal control and threatening to shoot the dog. I have heard of situations where neighbors have followed through with that threat.

Another friend moved because he hated his neighbor so much!

Disputes can occur over fences, trees, property lines, noise, etc. For my situation it was my trash cans.

Looking back, my situation borders on comical! My neighbor moved my trash can. Not a big thing, right? I mean I don't normally care where my trash cans are set out, but this became the sore spot for me and my neighbors. I probably need to say here too, that when I first moved into my house, my trash can was stolen! My ex-husband and I were in the middle of the divorce, so I thought the thief was probably trying to find dirt on me. Anyway, I never knew who took it, but it was gone – can and all!!! It became a joke every Thursday evening as I wondered if I would have a trash can when I woke up the next morning?! Lol

Here's where my trouble started. I had put the can out for trash pick-up when I left early that morning. It was in front of *my* property, yet as close as possible to my next door neighbor's house. I thought it was strange when I got home and my cans were on the opposite side of the driveway. I tilted my head and crinkled my brow, and thought it was strange, but simply put the trash cans back into the back yard.

The next week the exact same thing happened. I knew then that my next door neighbor seemingly did not like me leaving my trash cans on "his" side of my driveway. I was furious! The cans were in front of *my* property. They weren't in front of *his* property. How can he be mad about that? The third week I put the cans on the side closest to his property, and I was fully prepared to walk over and go ballistic on him, while explaining that he didn't have the right to tell me where to place my trash cans for pick-up as long as they were in front of my own property. The Lord reminded me that sometimes the best defense is silence.

Even a fool, when he holdeth his peace, is counted wise: and he that shutteth his lips is esteemed a man of understanding. Proverbs 17:28 KJV

It was at this point that I prayed for the Lord to be with me and to help me say the right words to my neighbor.

As I prayed I felt a check in my spirit. Hmmm. Yes, Lord??? Here was my inner battle:

Me: Maybe I should pray for my neighbor instead of yelling at him out for moving my trash cans.

God: What does my word say?
Me: Ummm. Count it all joy when you face trials of many kinds, because you know that the testing of your faith produces perseverance. Let perseverance finish its work so that you may be mature and complete, not lacking anything. .. James 1:2-8 (my version – lol)

God: What does my word say about neighbors?

Me: To love your neighbor.

God: Keep going…

Me: ...as yourself.

God: So what should you do?

Me: Put my trash cans on the other side?

God: You think?!

Me: (sheepishly) Yes...

> *Count it all joy when you face trials of many kinds, because you know that the testing of your faith produces perseverance. Let perseverance finish its work so that you may be mature and complete, not lacking anything... James 1:2-8 (my version – a blend of several)*

So I did. I began to count it all joy as I was putting my trash cans on the side furthest away from my neighbor's house. It was a simple solution. I fixed it. No cussing, no yelling at anyone, and in fact, no fighting at all. I just considered what I would want if I were my neighbor. I didn't have to be the mean neighbor. I had the power to turn this difficult situation around.

> *God can do more in one heart-receiving moment than we can do in a lifetime.*

I wasn't looking at the situation in a way where I had power. I wasn't looking at it from my neighbor's point of view. I was looking at it as if I were the victim of a neighbor that kept moving my trash can.

Later God showed me the scripture about going the second mile. The trash can wasn't where I wanted it. It was where my neighbor wanted it. Once I came to terms with what my neighbor wanted, I took back my own power! Someone once said:

Don't raise the bar. Be the bar!

So when someone hurts you or makes you mad, don't respond quickly. Never respond with vengeance. At first, just be silent. Pray for wisdom. Think about what Jesus would do. How would He want you to handle this situation? If you knew for a fact that this person would judge all Christians by your actions, what would you do? If you knew the only Bible this person would ever read or know about, would be to hear your words or see your response, what would you do? Then respond with Christ's love. It changes it, doesn't it?

> *By **this** shall all men know that ye are my disciples, if ye have love one to another.*
> *John 13:35 AKJV*

That alone will be a witness that you are a Christian. The Bible also says to be a peace with everyone if possible:

> *If it is possible, as far as it depends on **you**, live at peace with everyone.*
> *Romans 12:18 NIV*

With both of these scriptures, the onus is basically on *us*. We are not to show love ***if*** our neighbor shows love. We are to love anyway! We are not to be a peace with everyone ***if*** everyone is doing what we want. No! We are to be at peace if it's possible. Usually it's possible, because our personal will is involved.

I should add here that Duke's fight with his neighbor ended when he went to Walmart the day after Easter and bought a $1 basket that he filled with on-sale candy. He wrote an apology note and stuck it in the basket. He delivered and apologized in person. They now get along great. They even invited him to their 4th of July party! This works, folks!

Interestingly, those neighbors who moved my trash cans lived there for less than a year. They moved out and a wonderful couple moved in. They never once moved my trash cans! Ha! Ha! We get along great! I think sometimes we forget that God's ways are not *our* ways, but His ways are always better! So love your neighbor, keep the peace if possible, move your trash can, turn down your music, repair your fence so the dog can't get out, or do whatever you need to do for someone you live near, and don't forget to…

keep smiling…

If I say, 'I will forget my complaint,
I will change my expression,
and smile,..
Job 9:27 NIV

Chapter 16 – It's Not Easy to Keep Smiling

The struggle is real. It's not always easy to keep smiling. Life happens. It can chew you up and spit you out. Up until this point in my life, I thought I had experienced great difficulty. I had lost my best friend, my grandfather to a drunk driver, my other grandfather, and numerous friends. My grandmother has passed away and a week later I lost my dad. My mother and her mom, my other grandmother, died on the same day. My son was gay. My husband decided he wanted a newer, younger, skinnier wife. Hey, I was well-versed in loss and difficulty, or at least I thought I was.

When my husband had an affair and decided he did not want to work it out with me, I experienced loss in such a new and profound way. I just knew it couldn't get any worse. Then, as if on cue, his parents decided to throw me out of the family and acted as if *I* had done something wrong. It was not a time for smiling. His parents, who were also my pastors, determined they wanted no relationship with me or the grandchildren who were living with me. Talk about painful. It was intense. Like no other hurt I had endured previously.

Dan had even told me that he would be my dad when my father passed away (see page 34). Being treated like a stranger from those who had been my close-knit family and inner circle was unbearable. I could not understand why I was being treated this way.

I truly thought they would be on my side and at least attempt to help me try to keep my marriage together. At every turn, they disappointed me. I felt my children were also let down in their reaction. The church people were seeing how they reacted, and they, too, were not happy. I think everyone was anticipating them to react and respond in the way that they had preached about for 37 years, yet it didn't come. They continued down this path.

Don't get me wrong, I understood their love and compassion for Mike because I have 2 sons. I knew they would continue to love their son and support him. I just thought that they would also stand by me and continue to love me. The awful feeling of knowing they no longer wanted anything to do with me, was heartbreaking. I felt they threw the baby out with the bath water – exactly what my father-in-law had preached about *not* doing!

Yet, each day the sun came up. Each day there were things to be happy about. Yes, I could concentrate on the situation and be sad. However, most days I just kept repeating, "Lead on, Lord." I knew I was in His hands. I knew this was not the road I had planned to be on at this point in my life. I also knew that God would bring good out of it. So, step by step and breath by breath, I moved forward. I wasn't happy because my husband was no longer there. I was happy because Jesus Christ came into this world to save… me.

All I could do was be still and wait for Him to show me what to do next.

> *…stand still and see the Salvation of the Lord, which He will accomplish for you today." Exodus 14:13 NKJV*

I knew things that were working for my good…

And we know that all things work together for good to those who love God, to those who are the called according to his purpose. Romans 8:28-29 NIV

… and I knew life was good. I stayed busy with the two different Foundation Boards I was on. I continued playing the piano for the choir and the Chapelaires. I sang on the Praise Team. I babysat my precious little grandson as often as possible. I stayed busy with the kids. I allowed Sesily to have friends over to swim and hang out. It was what was best for me and for her – to keep life as normal as possible. I had the desire to entertain and have relationships. That old me that only saw fog (see page 106) walked out the door with my ex!

Perhaps God wants you to bloom where you find yourself planted – even if it feels like you're under cement at the moment. We have all seen a plant or a weed come up through concrete? It's amazing. If that is you right now, have faith. Look around. See what the work of the kingdom might be in your current situation - yes, even in a horrible situation! Maybe the current situation is going to be part of your future ministry. Has your child been sent to prison? Maybe you need to start a prison ministry and keep smiling. Has your home been leveled by a tornado? Perhaps you need to begin advising others who are going through the same thing. Has your spouse just left you for a younger version? Consider counseling those who are going through this painful path. Have you just received a terminal diagnosis? Start a prayer group that specifically prays for physical healing and keep smiling. Don't waste the opportunities you are given!

This path isn't where you had hoped to be at this point, but you're on this roller coaster, so throw up your hands and enjoy the ride!

I heard Bishop T. D. Jakes say to volunteer at the church or in the community ***even if*** you don't feel like it. Studies have shown that doing something good with the wrong attitude has benefits. We must remember that God is right here in the middle of our problems and difficulties. He's the God of the Mountain and the God of the Valley. The Hebrew meaning of the Alpha and the Omega includes everything in between. We often want to focus on the mountaintops or the valleys, but don't forget those times in between that may seem insignificant. It's important. Maybe it's the most important, because life if mainly lived in this "in-between" space.

Years later, Matt Nelson explained it in his book, *The Beauty of the In-Between*:

> *"Here is a simple, yet profound truth. When your eyes are set only on the destination, you miss everything that happens on the journey! Not just the difficult moments, but also and especially the beautiful moments. You're so locked in or driven or passionate that you miss life, you miss the people right in front of you, and you miss the beauty of God's goodness that can be found in everything. I'm learning to stop, to be present with the people I love the most, and to give them my very best. I'm learning that slowing down brings life. I'm learning that pausing and truly enjoying the moment makes all of life just a little bit sweeter." -Matt Nelson*

Here I was in the most difficult season I had ever been in, yet I also had some absolutely beautiful things happen. The summer of 2006, we went on several trips. Looking back, it is remarkable. I was unsure how much money I would end up with after the divorce, so I was being extremely careful how I spent. I was still living in our 6,000 square foot house and it was expensive to maintain without Mike's income. I also wasn't sure how long I would be living there, so I had to save money just in case it took several months. The Lord, however, always provided.

Sesily and I had one trip to Florida with some dear friends from church, which Mike was supposed to be on with us. The two of us went anyway! Our only cost was my round trip flight and Sesily's one way flight home because she rode there with them! I happily bought their dinner one evening, because they had paid for the condo, the rental car, the yacht, and all the other food! It was delightful.

Their condo overlooked two different angles of the bay at Punta Gorda. Almost every evening the dolphins would swim in, chatter, play, and entertain us. The pool for the condo was absolutely beautiful. The sunsets were spectacular. Then the *piece de resistance* was the yacht they rented for all of us! I truly felt like Jackie Kennedy riding in the back of Aristotle Onassis' yacht. Apparently I was born for this!

As we boated around, dolphins were jumping in and out of our boat's wake! We got some video of it and it was one of the most amazing experiences of my life! We took the yacht to the original Cheeseburgers in Paradise Restaurant on Cabbage Key. The ceilings and walls were covered with dollar bills! People had written their names and where they were from on the bills and tacked them up, so we had to join in the fun! The menu explained how when the dollar bills fall down, they donate them. So cool! The food was amazing and it was such a unique place. We all loved it!

When you are in the middle of something terrible, change your scenery. If you do, it makes it difficult to be thinking about your circumstance. Your mind is suddenly on what you are seeing and what you are doing. We enjoyed great food, fun, and fellowship. We played games, enjoyed nature, and chatted. It was exactly what Sesily and I needed. Thank you my friends, you know who you are!

In July we went on the youth Summer Safari. I went as a chaperone to help the youth group. It ended up being more of a blessing for me than I was for them! I talked almost the entire bus ride from Oklahoma City to Houston with another sponsor. It was a great time of fellowship. He truly ministered to me that day. He had read a book which had a lot to say about men and adultery. His insight was amazing and needed.

When we arrived at the hotel that night, I received a text message to go to the youth pastor's room to get something. We chatted for a bit and finally I returned to my room. The girls had filled the room with balloons and streamers for my birthday. I was turning 50! I had even received a text message from my ex earlier in the day. It seemed odd that he would be thinking of me, when it was apparent to me and everyone that he thought so little of me. Anyway, the girls filled my birthday with balloons, fun, well wishes and love! It was exactly what I needed! We had a fun trip! The youth group didn't get to do all of the events that were planned because it rained and the city of Houston flooded! It was still a blast, in spite of our plans being derailed by an unseasonable deluge of rain!

The Wednesday before this trip, the choir and dear friends hosted a surprise birthday party for me. I didn't know anything was going on. I walked into the welcome center and wondered why my children and grandchild were there. There were signs hanging from the ceiling, each with a word starting with an 'f' word to describe me, for example, fabulous, fun, feisty, fearless, flirty, etc. They had cake and also gave me cards. They had all donated and had a big balloon full of cash!!! I had never seen anything like it! As I've said, I was worried about my finances, so this was a perfect gift for me at the time. It was a great evening and reminded me that even if my ex didn't love me anymore, I *was* loved!!! This was a Godwink at a time when it was very needed. Urban Dictionary describes 'Godwink' like this: "An occurrence so odd and out of the ordinary, it had to be put in place by God. A wink from God letting you know you're moving in the right direction." Those 50 'f' words were exactly what I needed, more than the cash! They reminded me of my inner goodness and personality. I went home thankful and blessed, and full of the goodness of God and friends.

Later in July, we went on another trip. We had paid a $1000 deposit in January of 2006 for what we didn't know would be our final family vacation to Angelfire to ski but there was no snow. We continued on to Breckenridge, Colorado, where there was snow, to ski. My $1000 deposit was non-refundable and the hotel had made me choose a week that we would come back. I randomly chose my birthday week in July to return. I totally forgot about this until I received an email that they were expecting us to come! So Duke, my daughter, her best friend Megan, and I loaded up the car and drove to Angelfire for a week. We had no idea what to expect.

The condo was nice. We drove in to the town of Taos a couple of times, shopped, and saw a couple of movies. We played cards and games each evening. The rooms weren't air conditioned so all the windows were open. We could even hear bears getting into the trash at night. The town is pretty much dead in the off season.

We did go on an ATV tour. It was a blast but we got so dirty! In the funny pictures our faces are brown with dust, but very white where the goggles covered our eyes. Our rears were sore! All in all it was a blast.

Keeping busy and having fun kept us from thinking about our issues at home. When I went to check out, the woman said I had a credit from my initial deposit - it turns out rooms are much cheaper during July than during ski season, duh! She asked if I would like to put the extra back on my credit card. I hope I did not show the look of shock that was on my face! I shook my head yes, took my receipt and headed to the car. When I got home and figured up the cost of our meals, gasoline, etc., it was a few dollars short of my refund. It cost nothing to go on that little trip! God took care of me. Another Godwink!

The Lord had previously blessed us with a fun trip two months after I discovered the affair. Three of my dear friends – Tracy Loomis, Jodie Usry, and Lori Pipkin – two of which play and sing on our praise team took me, Sesily, and her friend Lindsay, to Branson. We didn't pay for one thing! We ate at great restaurants, saw shows, swam in the indoor pool, shopped, played miniature golf, had amazing conversations and even some middle of the night prayers together. The Lord knew I needed this!

Another group of my closest girlfriends, Becky Garland, Nikki Cheatham, and Lisa Garrett, took us to Lake Texoma for a week of scrapbooking and fun! We swam, grilled fantastic food, watched movies, read, quilted, cried, and talked until late at night! We laughed until my sides hurt. Mostly, we would reminisce about funny situations we had gone through together. We also went to the Lake Eufaula with my sister, Terri and family. We went boating, swam, picnicked, ate great food, watched movies, sat on the beautiful patio, drank morning coffee watching the sun come up, went on long golf cart rides, went tubing, and again – long talks. I even went fishing and with my brother-in-law's help, caught my first fish at 50 years old!

My broken heart was being internally stitched back together through each conversation and memory. So even though it was one of the darkest times in my life, every day the sun came up and every day was a good day. People would call at times when I was down. Terri and Vicki, my sisters, were a wonderful source of support. Good friends would invite me to do fun things to take my mind off of circumstances. People were praying for me throughout this entire situation.

If the Lord taught me anything through this first summer as a single woman, it was that friends are one of the most important things in our lives. Yes, my relationship with my husband and in-laws were important, but true friends are a gift. Scripture says it like this:

Friends come and friends go, but a true friend sticks by you like family. Proverbs 18:24 MSG

So keep your friends close, change your surroundings, get busy doing something good even when you don't feel like it, say yes when invited to go somewhere or do something, but most importantly…

keep smiling…

**God, your God,
is leading the way;
he's fighting for you.
Deuteronomy 1:30 MSG**

Chapter 17 – Nevertheless

Throughout my life, there have been times I prayed for God to intervene and he didn't. It was upsetting and sometimes sad. I have unquestionably had my fair share of unanswered prayers. Looking back, however, I got what I needed and not what I wanted.

This is exactly the place where some people lose their belief in a good God. They walk away from their Christianity. They figure God doesn't love them. God has forgotten them. Perhaps they think they haven't "performed" like God wanted them to. It is here, in the dark troubled time that we must truly trust Him.

When a child plays in the street, we don't allow it. They may kick and scream and say that is the best place to ride their bicycle, but we know best. We force them to stay out of the street for their own good. We can see what would or could happen if we allow it. It's the same with our heavenly Father.

I sometimes jokingly say that I'm a "spoiled brat." I don't know about you, but I want what I want when I want it. I am not patient. Here's a story about not getting what I wanted.

I believe it was in June of 2006: Dan-Dan called me yesterday and I called him back. It was probably the nicest call I had received from Dan or Bonnie since this whole thing started. Dan said he and Bonnie have been "trying to decide what to do about church." He said he wanted to take Sesily & I out to eat at Mazzio's - Sesily's favorite - tonight or tomorrow after church. I told him we were out of town, but we would love to very soon. He also said they are trying to plan a vacation. He explained that the board wanted him to take a couple of months off. He asked if we would go. I told him if anyone wants to take us anywhere, we're available. I said, "Our bags are packed and by the door." He laughed and said they missed us and wanted us to be a family again. He said, "We love you guys." I told him we had missed them and loved them too! I was in shock, but also so happy. It was very sweet and meant a great deal to me.

I had been waiting for this type of reaction since March. I actually thought maybe we had turned a corner here and things would be different. My prayer was to be able to have a great relationship with Dan and Bonnie, in spite of everything with Mike, and without Mike.

Silly, silly me.

I was about to be thrown out with the bathwater.

The next day or two, I talked to Mike's sister and found out that Dan and Bonnie were furious with me. They had received 3 letters: one from Tracy Loomis, one from Dana Covert, and one that was anonymous. They, of course, assumed I was behind all of them. Funny thing was, I had no earthly idea about any of them. Anyway, all the talk of a vacation trip and love and wanting to go to dinner, was immediately washed away. My prayers of having some sort of relationship with the family pretty much evaporated.

Looking back, although it was painful, it was probably for the best. I believe it would have been more difficult to stay in a relationship with them. I needed to separate from the entire family. It was excruciating. It was not what *I* wanted. It was what I needed. Isn't that just like Jesus? We are told in scripture:

God, your God, is leading the way;
he's fighting for you.
You saw with your own eyes
what he did for you in Egypt;
you saw what he did in the wilderness,
how God, your God, carried you
as a father carries his child,
carried you the whole way until you arrived here.
But now that you're here,
you won't trust God, your God –
this same God who goes ahead of you
in your travels to scout out a place to pitch camp,
a fire by night and a cloud by day
to show you the way to go.
Deuteronomy 1:30-33 MSG

Scripture also says in James:

You lust and do not have.
You murder and covet and cannot obtain.
You fight and war.
Yet you do not have because you do not ask.
James 4:2 NKJV

Yet, I asked and didn't receive the answer I wanted. I got the answer I needed. It can be confusing to a Christian. If your child is sick and you pray for healing, but then it doesn't happen – who can explain that away? No parent "needs" that. That is when you are forced – involuntarily required - to trust Jesus and know that somehow and some way, in eternity, you will come to understand why something like this happened.

I know of many who prayed to marry someone and years later they realized it would never have worked. They wouldn't have met their current spouse or had the children they have. Even Garth Brooks has a song called, "Unanswered Prayers." Here are part of the lyrics:

Sometimes I thank God
For unanswered prayers
Remember when you're talkin'
To the man upstairs
That just because he doesn't
Answer doesn't mean he don't care
Some of God's greatest gifts are
Unanswered prayers.
-Garth Brooks

So God was taking care of me – even when He wasn't answering my exact prayer. This is a very tough lesson to learn. It is hard to go through. This is where the rubber meets the road. My friend, Marla Lucas, who is on the radio in Springfield, Missouri, says it like this, "Life is about how well you handle Plan B!"

It's the truth. Sometimes it seems God is ignoring you. Maybe you believe God is mad at you. Maybe you are mad at God. Maybe He didn't answer your prayer. Maybe He let you down. Maybe you trusted Him and nothing happened. Maybe you've been patient and have had faith, yet He is still silent. Maybe you believe you have let God down. Pastor Kelly Roberts says,

"You don't have to worry about letting God down,
because you weren't the one holding Him up!"
- Kelly Roberts of Faith Uncensored Ministry

God is so easy to trust when He's answering prayers the way we want Him to. The real test comes when He isn't.

God, don't shut me out;
Don't give me the silent treatment, O God.
Your enemies are out there whooping it up,
the God-haters are living it up;
Psalm 83:1-2 MSG

The real test comes in His silence. Joseph kept trusting God, even in the pit, even in prison, even when the years slowly passed by. Max Lucado says in his book, *You'll Get Through This* (and some of it, I'm paraphrasing):

"God sees a Joseph in you. Yes, you in the pit. You with your family full of flops and failures. You, incarcerated in your own version of an Egyptian jail. God is speaking to you. Your family needs a Joseph, a courier of grace in a day of anger and revenge. Your descendants need a Joseph, a sturdy link in the chain of faith. Your generation needs a Joseph. There is a famine out there.

Will you harvest hope and distribute it to the people? Will you be a Joseph? Trust God. No, really trust Him. He will get you through this. Will it be easy or quick? I hope so. But it seldom is. Yet God will make good out of this mess. That's His job."
-Max Lucado

So, do you trust Him? Can you trust Him in your time of not understanding what is happening and why it is happening in your life? This is the struggle.

It's easy to talk about when you're not in the middle of it. It's easy to say you will trust God no matter what, but when the chips are down, can you? I think the better question is: Will you trust Him? It is an act of will.

Sometimes we know God is capable of doing something, but will He choose to?

I heard this and loved it:

> *"Hope doesn't go to sleep just because it's dark outside. It lights a candle and stays up, waiting for the rest of the story. Are you living in anticipation of God surprising you?*
> *This is the place where God meets us.*
> *It's in the power of the resurrection,*
> *the dark places. He finds us in the places between the miracles." – Bob Goff*

You need to realize that this is a precarious place to be. You must keep your eyes on the Lord. The chaos around you will someday stop. Remembering that in the middle of it all is hard. My kids and I have a favorite meme and gif. It shows a guy sitting at the kitchen table and the house is on fire. He is saying, "I'm fine. Everything is fine." Obviously for him, things aren't fine! We know, however, everything is *going* to be fine.

> *David said it all:*
> *I saw God before me for all time.*
> *Nothing can shake me; he's right by my side.*
> *I'm glad from the inside out, ecstatic;*
> ***I've pitched my tent in the land of hope.***
> *I know you'll never dump me in Hades;*
> *I'll never even smell the stench of death.*
> *You've got my feet on the life-path,*
> *with your face shining sun-joy all around.*
> *Acts 2:25-28 MSG*

I think it is okay to recognize that everything is *NOT* fine. Yet there needs to be faith that even though we can't currently see it, God will work it for our good. We need to have hope that everything is going to work out for our best! That is faith. I don't want you to be in denial for the trouble. I just want you to do what David did and pitch your tent in the land of hope.

Let me repeat that. Pitch your tent in the land of hope! You perhaps can't see things are going to get better, but if you have a tent in that land you can head that direction!

Looking back, it was a rough time. Here I was in the most difficult season I had ever been in, yet I also had some absolutely beautiful things happen. The summer of 2006, we went on several fantastic trips. However, if the devil can convince you that God chose not to answer your prayer, you may lose your faith altogether. Beth Moore says it like this:

> *"Faith is not believing in my own unshakeable faith. Faith is believing an unshakeable God when everything in me trembles and quakes."*
> *-Beth Moore*

This is why it is so important to believe *even* when things aren't turning out like you thought they would. Because of the Bible, I think as Christians we often think we know how God will want things to turn out. In my case, I figured I *KNEW* what God would want. After all, the Bible says in Malachi 2:16,

> *"I hate divorce," says the God of Israel.*
> *God-of-the-Angel-Armies says,*
> *"I hate the violent dismembering of the*

'one flesh' of marriage." Malachi 2:16 MSG

So with this knowledge, I just knew God would want to restore my marriage and my family. I prayed that Mike would come to his senses and that would happen. It didn't. Thankfully, I ended every prayer with…

NEVERTHELESS

This word has the ability to change any situation in any direction. It leaves all the power to God. It is a word that concedes power or authority or desire for an outcome and gives it back to God. Nevertheless is used 237 times in the Bible. Merriam-Webster says, it means, "However; in spite of."

In other words it says to God, however, in spite of my previous prayer, do what ***You*** *will.*

I knew what *I* wanted. In my heart and in my mind, I thought I knew what God wanted, however, in spite of that, I had to concede my desire for whatever God had for me. Here are a couple of scriptures that say the same:

And he went a little further,
and fell on his face, and prayed, saying,
O my Father, if it be possible,
let this cup pass from me:
nevertheless
not as I will, but as thou wilt.
Matthew 26:42 KJV

He went away again the second time,
and prayed, saying, O my Father,
if this cup may not pass away from me,
except I drink it, thy will be done.

Luke 23:34 KJV

Sometimes we are standing on the precipice of something amazing that we are afraid to step out into the unknown and into what God has for us. Circumstances can overwhelm you. It can be the most frightening time of your life. The fear of what's next is usually negative in our minds. Remember, however, God sees it all. This might be the most positive thing you have received yet!

Don't get too comfortable in your pity party! Don't give up in the middle of your battle. Don't do it! Don't give in! Remember God can open any door, even a back door. It may feel like you are leaving something behind that you love, nevertheless, if it is meant to be, God can open it again!

Pitch your tent in the land of hope.

Trust me when I say, I know this may be the most difficult situation you have ever gone through, **nevertheless**…

keep smiling…

But seek ye first the kingdom of God,
and his righteousness;
and all these things shall be added unto you.
Matthew 6:33 KJV

Chapter 18 – Sometimes You Get What You Need

Sometimes God doesn't give you what you want, but rather He gives you what you need. God wants you blessed. He wants you to be happy. Have you ever noticed though that what you thought would make you happy, doesn't bring you the happiness you thought it would?

Here are some notes from an Andy Stanley sermon that I watched on April 2, 2017, and I forgot to write the title:

God created the capacity for pleasure and happiness for humans. Happiness ultimately leads to pleasure. However, if you pursue pleasure or ignore the principles that lead to happiness, you will have neither. Eventually, pleasure loses its pleasure and becomes a prison. If any pleasure becomes your master, it becomes a prison.

Romans 6:16 - Don't you know that when you offer yourself to someone as obedient slaves, you are slaves of the one you obey - whether you are slaves to sin which leads to death, or to obedience, which leads to righteousness.

Sin always kills. Obedience to God offers yourself to peace with God which paves the way to peace with ourselves and equips us to make peace with others which equals happiness.

Happiness is not immediate. It must be sown. Following Jesus will make your life better. Ultimately you will reap.

Is there a pleasure that is undermining your happiness?

-Andy Stanley

Happiness is not immediate. It must be sown. Sown means, "to plant seed for growth especially by scattering." So to sow something means time is involved. That is often the hardest part. You can't plant an orange tree and expect a crop of oranges the next day. Water, sunlight, good soil, and care are all involved in the sowing of the orange tree seed. Time is also involved and it creeps by if you are waiting for an orange. We are like that. We want to be happy now!

Humans think that certain things will make us happy, but it never works. Once we get what we thought would make us happy, we are on to what we want next. We often barter with God saying things like, "God, if you give me what I want, then I'll go and do what you want." God actually works in the opposite direction. God says, "Go and do then I will give you what you need."

This is hard for most of us. We want God to do his part, then we'll do ours. However scripture says:

But seek first his kingdom and his righteousness, and all these things will be given to you as well. Matthew 6:33 NIV

I know too many people who have believed that they knew what they wanted and it would make them happy. Maybe they wanted a new house or a new car. Maybe they thought having a child would change everything for the better. Maybe they thought a different relationship would make them happy. Craig Groeschel says, "God never said, 'Be happy as I am happy.' Pastor Craig says, "God doesn't care if we are happy or not. God called us to be HOLY as He is holy."

I believe being holy will ultimately bring you the happiness you desire. We must seek first God's kingdom and THEN all these things – the happiness, peace, joy, love, contentment, etc. – will be given to you as well. I find it interesting that the attributes known as the fruits of the spirit use the term fruits. I just said earlier that we must sow our way to happiness. Fruit doesn't appear quickly. We must wait. The fruits of the spirit must be sown in our lives. We must seek first His kingdom and over time, the fruits will be revealed in our lives.

If I have any gardeners reading this, you know exactly what I'm talking about. You cultivate, plant, water, and care for your crop. You allow time to pass. You allow the dirt to do its work (stated in chapter 1). It may even seem like nothing is happening, but then one day you see something pushing up through the ground. Weeks later there is a small plant. Over time the plant grows and when you least expect it, fruit, or whatever you planted, is there waiting to be pulled from the vine!

Most people go through life thinking that the next big thing will make them happy. They are almost always wrong. Andy Stanley also says,

"Happiness depends on a 'who,' not a 'what.'"

Things never make us happy. We get one thing and immediately we move on to what "thing" we want next.

Seize life! Eat bread with gusto,
Drink wine with a robust heart.
Oh yes – God takes pleasure in your pleasure!
Dress festively every morning.
Don't skimp on colors and scarves.
Relish life with the spouse you love
Each and every day of your precarious life.
Each day is God's gift!
It's all you get in exchange
For the hard work of staying alive.
Make the most of each one!
Whatever turns up grab it
and do it. And heartily!
This is your last and only chance at it,
For there's neither work to do
Nor thoughts to think
In the company of the dead,
where you're most certainly headed.
I took another walk around the neighborhood
and realized that on this earth as it is –
The race is not always to the swift,
Nor the battle to the strong,
Nor satisfaction to the wise,
Nor riches to the smart,
Nor grace to the learned.
Sooner or later, bad luck hits us all.
Ecclesiastes 9:7-11 MSG

The scripture says sooner or later bad luck hits us all. The Amplified says in that same scripture, "…time and chance overtake them all." No matter how holy you are or how skillfully you are seeking first God's kingdom, bad luck hits us all. Another way to put that is from Matthew:

> *For he gives his sunlight to both the evil and the good, and he sends rain on the just and the unjust alike. Matthew 5:45b NLT*

To be happy *now*, it might be easier to disobey God. Some people get caught up in what feels good or seems good at the moment. Robert Morris says:

> *"Satan tell us, 'It is more pleasurable to disobey God than to obey Him. Things are going to go better for you if you eat the fruit than if you don't. Sin is the solution. If you sin then you will have joy, peace and pleasure.' Those very things will cause us to lose our close fellowship with God. Adam and Eve enjoyed close harmony with God. He hadn't withheld anything from them. But when we sin, it damages the relationship and separates us from God."*
>
> *–Robert Morris from the book Frequency*

If you are in a time of wanting to seek pleasure and thinking *that* will make you happy, you probably need to be spending more time in the scriptures. Have you ever noticed that when you didn't get what you thought would make you happy, it didn't really make that big of a difference in your life or outlook?

Remember to thank God for the things that are good in your life. Don't meditate or spend too much time thinking about what you don't have. Thank God for what He has done for you in the past. We are taught to make memorials and remember what God had done. Let that be a reminder of what He can do for you in the future.

Whatever you are going through now, God can see you through. The Israelites forgot what God had done for them. Instead of praising Him for delivering them from the Egyptians with all the miracles of the plagues, the Passover of the death angel, and parting the Red Sea, they began to focus on what they didn't have. They began to look at their situation through a negative filter.

I know people who may be in a huge battle of some sort, yet they have a great attitude and are so much fun to be around. That's because their mind is on the positive things in their life. They look at everything God has done for them and they are grateful. They are a breath of fresh air and endless summer.

I know others who aren't even in a terrible circumstance, yet they have a terrible attitude and are no fun at all to be around! They are sadly focusing on their current wants or needs and how God hasn't come through yet. They can bring you down. I call them "Debbie Downer," like the gal on Saturday Night Live! I usually try to get away as quickly as I can. If I'm not careful, they can take me down with them.

I have a friend or two that I hesitate to ask, "How are you doing?" I know if I do, there will be a long tirade of all the terrible things currently happening in their lives. Instead, I choose to say, "It's so good to see you!" That way, they don't have the opportunity to go down that long and winding dark road.

I want to be that breath of fresh air! I want to be the one that leaves people smiling. I want to be that endless summer for someone who is downcast and needs lifting up. Consider the words you are speaking over yourself and your life. I never want to be Debbie Downer and neither should you. I don't want people to want to get away from me. I choose to focus on the positive things that God has done in my life. There are many! Have I had a few lemons? Absolutely, however, my lemonade tastes fantastic!!! Life is good!

So seek first the kingdom of God. Don't waste time thinking about what you don't have. Dwell on the goodness of God in your own life and while you're doing that…

keep smiling…

**God will give you
new life again
Micah 4:10 MSG**

Chapter 19 –
God Is Taking Care of Me

God is/was/has been/will be taking care of me! I couldn't choose which one to put because they are all true! As I read through the pages of this book, that is the constant. On the good days and the bad, He was right there, just as it says in Isaiah 9:6, being my counselor, my Mighty God, my Father, my comforter, my Prince of Peace, my healer, and my provider.

For a child is born to us,
a son is given to us.
The government will rest on his shoulders.
And he will be called: Wonderful Counselor,
Mighty God, Everlasting Father, Prince of Peace.
Isaiah 9:6 NLT

He has been like the definition for 'constant' in Merriam-Webster's dictionary: "marked by firm steadfast resolution or faithfulness…" The bottom line is, whatever you are going through, God will be there to help you through it. That is the constant. You just have to trust Him. Ask Him to lead on!

I realize that it's hard to enjoy the journey when you are smack dab in the middle of it! Looking back is when we get perspective, and realize how far we've come and how wonderful God has truly been through it all. You will never understand the difficulties of the storm until you are able to see the strength, power, and growth that have been developing inside of you as a result of what you went through in your time of trouble.

Don't concentrate on what you have lost. Don't waste the love you've been given on someone who doesn't want it. Don't waste your tears on someone who has chosen they don't love you anymore.

Sometimes it takes losing
what you're settling for,
to get you to
what God wants you to have.

Sometimes it takes certain things falling apart for better things to fall into place. Sometimes it takes the most difficult paths to lead you to the most beautiful place. Your current situation is not your final destination. Don't get discouraged.

Think of the butterfly. Perhaps God wants to turn you from the caterpillar into a beautiful butterfly, but it will take going through a difficult process.

'Process' definition: a natural phenomenon marked by gradual changes that lead toward a particular result.'

It will be a struggle. It will create change. It will not occur quickly. It is a process.

Talking about changing from a caterpillar to a butterfly – this requires action on our part. God will be there for us but He expects us to do our part. We have to determine where we want to go and then move away from where we are, so that we can get there. Most of us are not comfortable with change. We like the status quo. We know what to do. When we step out into the unknown, it can be scary.

If you are in this spot, here are some things to do during the process when you are struggling:

a. Realize what you do matters.
b. Have a servant's heart
c. Work toward an attitude of prayerful service
d. Fill your tank so you can fill others

Let's discuss each one of these to truly understand what you can do when you're in a difficult situation. Let's look at a.) – Realize what you do matters. Sometimes we think what we do doesn't matter. You may think it won't mean much in the scope of eternity. Stop telling yourself that! It does matter! Remember words are powerful. The power of life and death is in the tongue. Tell yourself that what you do matters! Keeping kids in the nursery matters. Teaching Sunday School matters. Being a greeter or a Sunday School teacher matters!

I also urge you to go to this website for encourage that what you do matters. Click here to listen to Andy Andrews' Butterfly effect:

https://search.yahoo.com/search?fr=mcafee&type=C211US885D20150813&p=andy+andrews+butterfly

In easy to understand language, the butterfly effect means that every small thing we do can impact someone or something. Get involved. Do what you can. Here is the Wikipedia explanation for it:

> *The butterfly effect or sensitive dependence on initial conditions is the property of a dynamical system that, starting from any of various*

arbitrarily close alternative initial conditions on the attractor, the iterated points will become arbitrarily spread out from each other.

Sometimes we are in circumstances that make us feel like we can't do anything that will make a difference. We may feel that the devil is currently controlling our life. That is not the case! Look at what the scripture says:

And I will deliver thee
Out of the hand of the wicked,
And I will redeem thee
Out of the hand of the terrible.
Jeremiah 15:21 KJV

Note the glorious personality of the promise. "*I*" will. The Lord puts himself in the middle of their trouble. He says *He* will personally rescue them. Notice there is nothing said of *our* effort needed to assist the Lord. Our strength is not taken into account. Our weakness is not discussed. The Lord says, "*I,*" will redeem.

Up until this, we've been talking about *our* part - what *we* do for the Lord, *but* we should always remember that He will do His part when it matters or when we've done all we can do!

Be diligent to present yourself approved
to God, a worker who does
not need to be ashamed,
rightly dividing the word of truth.
2 Timothy 2:15 KJV

We must be diligent. I also love that it tell us to

"...rightly divide the work of truth."

Nonbelievers often say that the Bible contradicts itself. It never does *IF* it has been rightly divided. True, we can take a scripture out of context and say that it goes against something else in the Bible. However, if we study and accurately and honestly study all of it, it does not contradict itself. We must study and not leave our beliefs up to others! When we are the one who has been diligent, God will use us and then we will be able to make a greater impact.

This leads me to another question and to **b.)** – Have a servant's heart. Has the Lord asked you to do something that you aren't doing? It is not my intent to place condemnation on you, but perhaps we should all think about this. We need to be working for Him to further His kingdom. Are you hungry to see God's kingdom expanded? Are you wanting God to do something in you so that he can do something through you?

He will gather the lambs with His arm.
Isaiah 40:11

In His flock there are a wide variety of experiences and backgrounds.

Some of us are strong in the Lord,
while others may be weak
either in faith or in ability.

Remember, Jesus is our Shepherd.

Jesus cares for all His sheep.
The weakest may be as precious to Him
as the strongest of the flock.

Lambs are known to be animals that are dependent on someone to show them where to go and what to do. They often lag behind, are prone to wander, or even grow weary at inopportune times. They depend solely on their Shepherd to keep them away from all the dangers of this world! The Shepherd makes sure the new-born lambs are fed. He watches over the young lambs. If he sees one about to perish from a predator, He does what He can to protect them. The Shepherd loves each one!

He watches over all of us, ready to rescue and keep from harm, even those who have gone astray! I believe if we do what we can, Jesus will help us to do what we need to do. He will open doors for us. He will do great and mighty things to help our small steps.

We also need to have **c.)** – work toward an attitude of prayerful service. If we just begin doing something but we haven't prayed about it or asked God what He wants us to do, then we will probably be spinning our wheels. I do think it is okay to work for the Lord in almost any capacity and He will bless it. I also believe, however, if you are truly doing what God wants you to, it will be more purposeful and more powerful.

God knows what He's doing. If we align ourselves with how best to serve Him, the outcome will be far greater than if we are just working to work. These two scriptures say it perfectly:

> *So, then, my friends,*
> *because of God's great mercy to us*
> *I appeal to you:*
> *Offer yourselves as a living sacrifice to God,*
> *dedicated to his service and pleasing to him.*

This is the true worship that you should offer.
Romans 12:1 GNT

and

So here's what I want you to do,
God helping you: Take your everyday,
Ordinary life – your sleeping, eating,
going-to-work, and walking-around life –
and place it before God as an offering.
Embracing what God does for you is the
Best thing you can do for him.
Don't become so well-adjusted
To your culture that you fit
Into it without even thinking.
Instead, fix your attention on God.
You'll be changed from the inside out.
Readily recognize what he wants from you,
and quickly respond to it.
Unlike the culture around you,
always dragging you down to
its level of immaturity,
God brings the best out of you,
develops well-formed maturity in you.
Romans 12:1-2 MSG

After my divorce, I looked back on those 30 years and felt they didn't make sense. I spoke to the district superintendent who told me that I "didn't work for the Assemblies of God." Mike had been a minister and I was "just his wife." I was shocked. I felt I had been working for the AG for 30 years, yet once again was being treated as if I were an outcast. So instead of getting offended and angry, I got busy and began the School of Ministry to get my own AG credentials.

Some people look for reasons to be offended and not participate. They sit on the sidelines talking about how no one is doing things correctly, and how much better it would be if they were in charge. I say to stop judging instead of participating. It is easy to not believe or to accuse others. If you are busy and involved, you won't have time for such petty things!

Some feel like they can't get involved because they aren't good enough or spiritual enough. They may still be living in sin. Just remember sin creates distance between you and God, but it doesn't create a diminishing of His great love for you! Go ahead and do what you can. Let God take care of the details. Generally people don't change so God will lead us to where we need to be. We change because God loved us! If you move forward, soon your priorities will align with His. That is the thing that proves the presence of God.

Last but certainly not least is **d.)** – fill your tank so you can fill others. I know that some of us in Christian church work, can be "spent" emotionally and spiritually, yet we keep showing up every Sunday. Don't get me wrong, that is admirable in today's world! However, we need to show up with a full tank. We need to be ready to pour ourselves out to those who are hungry. However, like me years ago, too many forget to fill their own tank before they come. Be sure you are spending time in the Word, listening to programming that will minister to you, attending church when you are soaking it in and not always ministering, etc. I suggest watching other churches online, going to conferences, and even visiting other churches. Last but not least, listen to Christian radio in your car, and sing at the top of your lungs, giving Jesus the highest praises!

These are all so important. I was involved in church work during a time that it was frowned upon to miss church or to not be at your post every Sunday. What I didn't realize was that my love tank for Jesus was getting lower. If my ex-husband and I had been diligent, we could have easily taken a break and filled our love tanks back up. It was too late for my marriage. However, by the time I did that, it was too low. I had let it get too low. I needed to completely refill. Take care not to get into that position. That is when Satan can come in and cause irreparable harm to your life, your relationships, and your ministry.

Take time off. Some churches now require staff to be away for a certain number of weeks. We could only miss 2 Sunday's per year. Looking back, it wasn't enough. I was told for many years that if I visited another church, I was somehow being unfaithful to my church. Now I feel differently. I feel I can go visit another church and receive spiritual food. I am not telling you to miss every Sunday, but I am suggesting that every once in a while, take some time away to renew and refresh yourself. When we fill ourselves to overflowing, that is when we can truly make a difference in someone else's life. If we are empty, we have nothing to give. Just like our cars. If our car has no gas, it can't take us to where we want to go. We must be filled with the Holy Spirit. We must be reading our Bible so that we can be used by the Lord.

The Lord is my shepherd; I shall not want.
He makes me to lie down in green pastures;
He leads me beside the still waters.
He restores my soul;
He leads me in the paths of righteousness
For His name's sake.
Yea, though I walk through the
valley of the shadow of death,
I will fear no evil; For You are with me;
Your rod and Your staff, they comfort me.
You prepare a table before me
in the presence of my enemies;

You anoint my head with oil;
My cup runs over.
Surely goodness and mercy shall follow me
All the days of my life;
And I will dwell
in the house of the Lord Forever.
Psalm 23 NKJV

So to review, doing these four things, helps us have responsibility and accountability in our lives:

a. Realize what you do matters.
b. Have a servant's heart
c. Work toward an attitude of prayerful service
d. Fill your tank so you can fill others

The Lord wants us to be one of His lambs, solely dependent upon Him. We get to decide whether we are a lamb or a goat. Remember lambs come when their master calls. They recognize His voice. Sheep have always been considered as the emblems of mildness, simplicity, patience, and represent the genuine Disciples of Christ. Sheep don't make their own decisions. They go where the master wants them to.

Goats are naturally quarrelsome, and ill-scented. Isn't that such a nice way of saying 'stinky?' lol Goats are considered symbols of comedy, and being profane and impure. Biblically, they often represent those who have lived and died in their sins. Goats do not come when they are called. They don't go where their master tells them. I see so many "goats" in our world today. The older I get, the more ready I am to see Jesus sort the people out, just as the Bible tells in Matthew that He is going to. I'm pretty sure I could help Him!

When he finally arrives,
blazing in beauty and all his angels with him,

the Son of Man will take his place
on his glorious throne.
Then all the nations will be
arranged before him and
he will sort the people out,
much as a shepherd
sorts out sheep and goats,
putting sheep to his right
and goats to his left.
Matthew 25:31-46 NIV

Now I don't know about you but I want to be a sheep. Psalm 23 says, "The Lord is *my* shepherd..." I want to be one of *His* sheep. I don't want to be a goat - a disobedient, stinky, smelly goat – doing selfish things. I want to be an obedient sheep that knows my master's voice, so that when Jesus calls for me, I'll come and I'll recognize His voice. If you want that to be one of His sheep, and turn your life over to Him, pray this prayer:

Lord, help me today to be your sheep. Teach me to hear your voice, even if I haven't listened to it in the past. Show me the way you want me to go. Keep me close to you. Come into my heart and give me the heart of a sheep, willing to trust you with my life. I don't want to be an unruly goat. I want the inheritance that you've set aside for me from the beginning, the inheritance that you intended for me from the foundation of the world. Help me to be in your perfect will. Help me to trust You, obey You, and love You better in this lifetime.

In Jesus name, Amen.

I hope you prayed that prayer and meant it. If you did, you have invited Jesus to rule your life. Jesus, our master, watches over all of us, ready to rescue and keep from harm, even those who have gone astray! I believe if we do what we can, Jesus will help us to do the rest. Your weakness can become your strength.

Your pain can become your power. Your confusion can become your peace. Your heart will heal. You mind will be clear. Your tears will dry. Your pain will end. Let the hard times of your life turn into the best times of your life. The "hurt" you can turn into the "greatest" you! What you have been going through will eventually be everything you made it through!

Just because something is over,
doesn't mean your life is over!

Today is a new day, a new beginning. What do YOU want to do? Where do YOU want to go? What have YOU always wanted to do, but never had the time or the opportunity to do? See yourself as equipped and empowered. What do you need from the Lord? He will give you what you need. He will take care of you, if you trust Him and if you let Him. He will open doors for you. He will do great and mighty things to help your small steps.

And while you're taking those small steps, remember to…

keep smiling…

Chapter 20
God Will Give You New Life Again

So here I am, many years down the road from some of my worst life experiences. Some may look at me and think I have gotten over them. I would say you never really get over them, but you do get through them. They are always with you, but have become more of a reminder of what God can do rather than what He can't do.

Each experience I encountered is different and God ministered to me in different ways. When my friend left for Africa, God provided the piano to get me through. When my parents passed away, I had church work and mission work in Africa to attend to. When my son came out about his sexuality, my own belief in God's word was put to the test, yet once again God met me there.

When my ex-husband decided he didn't want to work it out with me, I felt my very foundation had been rocked. We had been a team; a good team. I typically explain it as someone who has lost their right arm. At first I didn't think I could do anything. Everything was new, challenging, and difficult. Soon, I got pretty good at navigating a different life without a husband. Yes, it was hard and yes, it was not without new problems I had to face. However, God's grace is sufficient.

It reminds of the man with the withered hand in Mark 3:1-6. I wonder if this man had lived in today's world, if he would have shown pictures on Facebook and Instagram of only his "good" hand. I have come to believe we must show our failures, our flaws, and our disappointments, for Jesus to be able to heal them. I know that once my dirty laundry was aired, I was able to help people and truly minister to people in a way that was impossible when I had what others viewed as a perfect life.

Yet in all these things we are
more than conquerors through
Him who loved us.
For I am persuaded that
neither death nor life, nor angels,
nor principalities nor powers,
nor things present nor things to come,
nor height nor depth
nor any other created thing,
shall be able to separate us
from the love of God
which is in Christ Jesus our Lord.
Romans 8:37-39 NKJV

I take this scripture to mean that *we* hold the power in our own hands whether we allow a situation to separate us from God. It won't happen to me, unless I let it. If you are someone who goes back and forth with your beliefs, maybe it's time you make a decision not to allow *anything* to get in the way of your relationship with God.

If you continually find yourself in the same terrible situation again and again, perhaps you need to look at yourself instead of blaming those around you. If you are divorced, remarried, struggling relationally, or are always losing your job or your friends, ask yourself what you could do differently. Truly reflect on your part.

> *I'm trying to say again – when*
> *life hands you lemons,*
> *make some lemonade!*

When life gives you a bad hand, don't fold! Don't give up and don't give in. Use it to start anew with a better attitude and more knowledge! Jesus told the man with the withered hand to "…stretch…" forth his hand. One of the definitions of 'stretch' is, "To go beyond what is strictly warranted in making a claim or concession." Another definition is, "an exercise of something, such as the understanding or the imagination, beyond ordinary or normal limits." Think about that. Jesus wants us to move beyond our ordinary or normal limits! Can we do that? I think we can, but only with His help!

God's grace is sufficient to see you through whatever awful time you are going through. The time in the valley, where you question everything, is often the time when God meets you, ministers to you, and heals your broken heart. The time between the dreadful circumstance you are in and the victorious mountain is fertile ground for God to work. God can show you things in the valley that you might never come to understand on the mountain top. It is a fruitful time for holding on to God in a new way.

I love what Matt Nelson says about those times in his book *The Beauty of the In-Between*:

> *"This 'theology of the in-between' is essential to understanding that waiting is not a waste. In fact, the waiting is when God does some of his best work and our*

level of faith is elevated to the next level. Faith is not always necessary when we're living in the miracle or the fulfillment of the promise, but faith becomes a premium when we can't see the end result".
– Matt Nelson from the book The Beauty of the In-Between

I don't care who you are, at some point in your life, you will be put through a tremendous difficulty. I gave you the scriptures earlier explaining it happens to us all. We might question whether we did something to bring us to this place, or perhaps you had nothing to do with. Maybe a tornado has hit your home. Maybe you have been unable to get pregnant. Maybe you have truly sought and put God's kingdom first and foremost, and yet you find yourself with a terminal diagnosis. Do you deserve this? Usually the answer is no.

As crazy as it sounds, this is part of life. We live in a sinful world where bad things happen. It places us in a sort of wilderness that can even feel like God has forgotten us. Our prayers aren't being answered. Our situation is bleak. Where is the God of salvation and rescue? Sometimes He leaves you right there in that place of darkness, like a big holding tank.

The waiting and the place where all prayers go unanswered is, as I've mentioned before, where real trust begins. My advice is to hang on! Tie a knot in the end of your rope and hang on! Do not give up hope!

Do not turn from your faith, turn toward it.

Do not let go of your dreams! So many abandon the call God placed on their lives during this time. The devil tries to get you to doubt everything! He works hard to make you believe that if it hasn't happened, then it isn't going to happen.

Matt Nelson also says in *The Beauty of the In-Between*,

> *"Learning to embrace God's process,*
> *His bigger picture for life,*
> *Will require us to take a*
> *Huge step of faith.*
> *The waiting will require us*
> *To master everything we know*
> *To be true about who God is!"*
> *-Matt Nelson*

Wherever you are on your journey, focus on what you have and not what you have lost. Many lose their way because they focus on what they've lost or might lose. Stay positive! Be the star in your own life! Dr. Phil always has good sound advice and he says it like this:

Star in your own life!
Drink it in.
Success is a succession
Of moments, so don't miss it.
-Dr. Phil

We often want to hide the terrible things that happen in our lives. We want to show the highlight reel of only the good things on social media. We love to spotlight the times when everything is good. That is ***not*** how God works. The pain that you have suffered will be a tool to draw others to you.

The man with the withered hand in Mark 3 was not ashamed to show his hand. If the man had been hiding his problem, Jesus may not have healed it. The man, however, apparently made no attempt to hide it, thus it was restored and made whole.

As I look back on my life with 20/20 vision and a new perspective, I realize that my mess *has* become my message which was my prayer in the beginning of my mess with my former husband. I speak with men and women all the time, who have been betrayed and whose spouses have been unfaithful, whose children have come out of the closet, whose lives have been turned upside down by a death of a close family member, or many others issues. I believe people feel comfortable coming to me because they know that, like Jesus, I am acquainted with pain. They know I've walked through the fire and with Jesus' help have come out the other side without even the smell of smoke. Your pain is what attracts others to you.

The redeeming qualities of Christ are that He takes what was the mess and wreckage of our lives, and redeems it by helping someone else who is going through the same thing. When this happens, all of a sudden, every painful situation has a purpose. Every horrible pain you have suffered has been exchanged for someone else's lesson and encouragement. That is true redemption. Your pain for someone else's gain. Isn't that just like Jesus? He suffered for our gain.

Years ago I remember reading Rick Warren's book, *The Purpose Driven Life,* thinking, "Duh, doesn't everyone know this?" I knew that even small things in our life mattered to God. I knew that our actions, big and small, are basically purposeful for the kingdom of God. Now that I look back over these past many years, I have learned that God uses the good times and bad times and the in-between times for His purposes.

Realizing God uses *everything* for His purposes, makes it all worthwhile. Terrible memories can become good, or at the very least, resolute in the good that has come from it. Looking back at the unpleasant situations, no longer needs to be painful and hurtful.

No matter what, your story does *not* end in defeat. If you have read the end of the Book, then you know you are victorious! Good will come of what you have suffered. If you have lost your dreams, or worse, your belief in God, it's time to begin trusting that He is in control – even if you don't fully understand it at the moment. He suffered so that we could have salvation.

> *He is despised*
> *and rejected by men,*
> *A man of sorrows*
> *And* ***acquainted with grief.***
> *And we hid, as it were,*
> *Our faces from Him;*
> *He was despised, and*
> *we did not esteem Him.*
> *Isaiah 53:3 NKJV*

The same scripture in The Message says,

> *He was looked down on*
> *And passed over,*
> *A man who suffered,*
> *Who knew pain firsthand.*
> *Isaiah 53:3 MSG*

Jesus knew pain firsthand. He has direct and personal experience to human pain, loss, abandonment, despair, and agony. He *knows* what you're going through. That, in itself, is comforting. Jesus wants to help you through whatever it is you are experiencing.

He knows how to help you because He went through it all – pain, loss, betrayal, agony, despair, abandonment.

He knows and He sees.

Invite Him into your pain. Show Him your withered hand. Ask for His direction as the master of your life. Become one of His sheep, allowing Him to guide and direct you.

I can say that it is true. The truth does set you free. The Bible says in John 8:32,

And you shall know the truth,
And the truth shall make you free.
John 8:32 NKJV

In other words, Jesus knows what you are feeling. Remember, He knows pain. No matter what you are suffering with - relationship problems, addictions, codependency, depression, boundaries or any other issues, Jesus can heal you. There is hope. Jesus can restore what is lost. If addicted to a substance or pornography, Jesus can help you change the cycles of insanity that plague your life.

Don't you want to be free from all the pain in your life?

First you must show Him your withered hand or whatever your problem is, by admitting and confessing your sin and what you need help with.

Have an honest and real conversation with Jesus. Tell Him what you need. Tell Him what you've been going through. Ask for the Holy Spirit to help you. Ask for supernatural strength to lay it all out on the line. I can guarantee, Jesus will meet you there.

You may feel like you have done too much to be forgiven. You may feel you are not worthy. You may feel you are too far gone. You may not be the person who has gone through all the pain, but perhaps you are the person who has caused all the pain. God will still be there when you are ready to ask for His forgiveness and help moving forward. You are not too far from God. Nothing could be further from the truth. If you step toward God, He will come running to you. Reread the story of the prodigal son. The father is simply waiting for your return.

The story of the prodigal son is found in Luke 15:11-32. It is a parable explaining the joy the Father God receives over every sinner who repents from the sin life they are currently living. In the story the father has two sons. One asks for his inheritance, which he soon wastes. This son finds himself living in a hog pen, and so he returns to his father hoping to live as a servant. As soon as the father sees him, he begins to run toward his son, throws his arms around him and kisses him. The story goes on to say, "But the father said to his servants, 'Quick! Bring the best robe and put it on him. Put a ring on his finger and sandals on his feet. Bring the fattened calf and kill it. Let's have a feast and celebrate. For this son of mine was dead and is alive again; he was lost and is found.'"

This parable has God as the Father and the sinner as the prodigal son. We may have squandered our opportunities with our heavenly Father, but in the end, it doesn't matter. God's grace is like the grace of the father in the story. He is simply happy to have his son, or daughter, home again. That's how God feels about you turning back to him. If you have turned away from

God or if you have just felt abandoned because He didn't answer your prayers, pray this prayer:

Dear Heavenly Father,

Thank you for the opportunity to come to you and ask for forgiveness. I have been experiencing great difficulty. I pray for help because of the things that I am going through. I don't understand and frankly, I am unable to see that any good will come from it. I ask that Jesus would be my personal savior. Give me peace. Give me wisdom. Draw me closer to You, and as I take each step, light my path and lead me, so I will know that You are good, and You are right here with me.

It's in Jesus' name I pray, Amen

If you prayed that prayer, then you have been born again. Now you can begin this new phase of your life, where you allow God to take control. Find a Bible believing church and begin attending every service. I have faith Jesus will be closer than a brother to you. You don't have to understand everything right now, but just begin the walk.

Doug Clay in the article *Spirituality and Missions* in the Assemblies of God's Influence Magazine states,

"We all want to experience the power of Christ's resurrection. But it's often in the fellowship of Jesus' sufferings that we draw closer to him and become more like him. It's in a difficult, desperate, lonely places that we reach the end of ourselves and discover more of him. If Christ is all we have, we quickly realize Christ is more than enough." -Doug Clay

This is so true. Whatever you're going through, Jesus will be there and He will be enough.

If you are already a Christian, but you are in the middle of some terrible turmoil, stand firm. In the prayer, you asked him to enter into your current troubles. We have to be like Jerimiah 17:7, 8 says,

Be like a tree
planted by the water which
spreads out its roots by the river,
and will not fear when heat comes;
Jeremiah 17:7-8 NKJV

Look at that scripture carefully. It doesn't say ***IF*** the heat comes but ***WHEN*** the heat comes! It is telling us right there tough times *will* come but don't fear and don't worry, because if your roots are deep in the Lord, you will be fine.

The three Hebrew children knew this. They came through the fire without even the smell of smoke. Glory! I know their faith must have been tested. Their roller coaster took a big scary dip down into a hot furnace. I know that they said their God would deliver them, but they had faith that ***even if*** God didn't, He must have a master plan and they were a part of that plan. Whatever you are going through and however horrible it may seem, it doesn't mean God doesn't have a plan for you. Sometimes when it seems the worst, you are exactly where God wants you to be.

We have to keep in mind there are times when pain brings something good. For example, childbirth, vaccinations, surgery, dental work (ugh - I had to throw that in there because just a few weeks ago I had the absolute worst dental experience of my life – ouch!!!). In the end it is worth it. Now while you're in it, it may not seem like it's worth it but it is. One day we'll look back with 20/20 vision and see that it was. We will see what God was doing.

If you are at a breaking point, it is here at that breaking point that God asks us to hold out - even when everything around us screams to give up. As I said before, even Jesus had his faith tested. When he was on the cross and his faith and endurance was stretched (there's that word again) to the breaking point and he cried out,

"My God, my God, why have you forsaken me?"

It's easy to trust God when things are going well. I ask that question again - can you trust God when things aren't going well?

God saw the outcome. He knew that in the end, it was going to be better. When I think of my savior, bloody and bruised and dying on that cross, yes I wish he didn't suffer… but I'm so glad He stayed up there. For me. For you. He hung on through the biggest dip of His roller coaster. He cried out, but he made it. God was allowing Jesus' pain for the greater good. He hung on… and because He did, it is finished. It is complete. We just have to do like He did and endure… and that can be hard. That can be a giant step of faith.

So in the end, the only event that should define your life is on a hill called Mount Calvary. If you know that, then everything else falls perfectly into place.

I don't just believe in Jesus or believe He is real. I know Him because He has walked with me through some incredibly painful things. He has also given me some incredible blessings. When we see as Jesus sees and understand as He understands, we will want to live as He wants us to live.

Years ago, I determined to live my life backwards as my mother did. She was doing this when I was a kid. I decided to do this long before there was a book about it. Each thing I did, was with a thought about what would be said at my funeral if I went through with it? It has been a moral compass. It has helped guide me to try to be the very best I can be in all circumstances in my life. In the end you are remembered for your actions. Now this doesn't mean that if you mess up, you'll be remembered for messing up. It simply means you'll be remembered for what you do after you mess up!

For over 30 years, I had always dreamed of a perfect family. When my family broke apart, I realized there were no perfect families in the Bible. I read the Bible with a different vantage point. Every story was messy. Even Jesus' family had issues. James, Jesus' brother, didn't become a follower until *after* the resurrection. I mean, who could deny that Jesus wasn't who He said He was when He rose from the dead? Apparently not James! Before that however, I picture James rolling his eyes every time his mother called Jesus the son of God! Ha!

However, in all the messy families, God was there. Scripture called Jesus, Emanuel which means God *with* us. In every difficulty, He was there. God said in Exodus 3:4-12,

"...but I will be with you..."

It's a promise.

When God is in it with you, you can do what you think you can't.

We can give in, give up,
or give it all we've got!

That is excellent advice if I do say so, myself! Give it all you've got! God will be right there beside you. He will lead you on. We often look for God in places that everyone recognizes, like church and funerals. However, God is often found in the trivial and lonely places of our lives. The two men on the road to Emmaus did not recognize the resurrected Jesus there because they weren't looking for him. They figured this remote road they were on was too unimportant. Even today guides in Israel are not positive that this is the actual road to Emmaus because it was inconsequential back then and hardly worth naming.

> *Perhaps Jesus chose to meet those two men there to demonstrate that He is the God of the insignificant journey from wherever you came from to wherever you are going.*

He's with you when you're walking the wrong way or with the wrong people. He's with you when you're walking the right way and life is good. He's with you when you're walking through disappointment or pain. In other words, He's with you.

He is not only beside you but He is also within you! So it doesn't matter what insignificant road you are on. He is there! It's about moving forward. It's about you meeting Jesus along life's road. It's about you letting Jesus lead.

No matter what has happened to you during your life, the redeeming Christ takes what was the wreckage of your life and exchanges it by helping someone else who is going through it. This all of a sudden makes it worthwhile, good, and happy, instead of painful.

As usual, it is our attitude that makes the difference. How are you viewing the difficulties that have come your way?

Are you making lemonade out of lemons, or are you wallowing in self-pity that life has been so cruel to you?

> *"We can complain because*
> *rose bushes have thorns,*
> *or rejoice because thorns have roses."*
> *-Alphonse Karr*

Somewhere in the past few years, I wrote a poem which speaks to me:

<u>To Matter</u>

All any of us really want is to matter.
But the only thing
that really does matter
is our relationship with God.
In the end who cares where you work
or what you wear
or how much money you have.
But do you know God?
Do you seek Him daily?
Do you read His word?
Are you still
and do you listen for His voice?
Would you know it if you heard it?
In the end what matters
is that you know Him.

I've heard it said that happiness is an inside job. I know that this is true. We must determine every day to get up, show up, and keep smiling. Is it hard sometimes? Absolutely! Is it worth it? Always!

I'm here to let you know that God's grace is sufficient. Through all the pain and all the hurt, God has been right there for me. I've had to lean pretty hard. Some of the days were so painful, it was excruciating. Yet here I am, whole, well, and healed. Ready to face the rest of my life with me… and I like me. I had forgotten how much I like Sandy. She is amazing! I'm so glad to have her back. I had been convinced me that I was the one lacking and I'm not.

I have a great life – one I wouldn't trade it for anything! My children and grandchildren bring me so much joy! I'm so thankful to have walked this journey with them. It has brought us a closeness that others talk about and want for their own. It was difficult and a process, but here we are!!!

You are amazing too! Don't forget that! Don't let the circumstances change your disposition. If you are a follower of Christ, then all that really matters is that you have salvation and will spend eternity in heaven because your name is written in the lamb's book of life. Everything else is temporary. You can handle it.

I have come so far that I am able to see my mess *is* now my message. I look out my window now and see so much more than fog. I see a bright future, full of hope and expectation. God is leading and guiding me every step of the way, every day.

All I have to do now is…

keep smiling!

THE END

Bibliography/Works Cited

Active Christiany, *19 Bible verses showing God's thoughts toward us*, https://activechristianity.org/19-bible-verses-showing-gods-thoughts-toward-us, Copyright 1982

Andrews, Andy. *The Butterfly Effect Video*. YouTube, 2013, https://video.search.yahoo.com/search/video?fr=mcafee&p=andy+andrews+butterfly#id=1&vid=bfa0cc9e57f3b7ef283769e846f94d14&action=click , Retrieved on July 26, 2020

Borques, Michelle, et al. Live, Laugh, Love Again ISBN 0-466-69609-9 New York, NY Warner Faith www.warnerfaith.com Copyright 2006

Chapman, Gary D. The Five Love Languages; ISBN 1-881273-15-6 Chicago, IL Northfield Publishing www.fivelovelanguages.com Copyright 1992, 1995, 2004

Clay, Doug. *Spirituality and Mission*. Assembly of God Influence Magazine. Issue 33. Jan-Mar 2021

Conway, Jim. Men in Midlife Crisis. ISBN 1-56476-698-5
1st printing revised edition 1997 Colorado Springs, CO Life Journey www.CookMinistries.com/LifeJourney. Copyright 1978, 1997

Cowman, L.B. Streams in the Desert. Zondervan Publishing. ISBN 978-031- 060-7052. Copyright 1925, 1953,1965, 1996, 1997

Edwards, Gene. A Tale of Three Kings; ISBN 0-8423-6908-2 Wheaton, Illinois; Tyndale House Publishers, Inc.; Copyright 1980, 1992

GotQuestions.org, *What does it mean that Jesus is the Alpha and the Omega?*, https://www.gotquestions.org/alpha-and-omega.html, Retrieved on June 11, 2020

Hagen, Kenneth. Love the Way to Victory, English. ISBN: 0892765232. ISBN13: 9780892765232. Release Date: July 1994. Publisher: Faith Library Publications, Incorporated. Copyright 1991.

Holy Bible, New Living Translation ®, copyright © 1996, 2004 by Tyndale Charitable Trust. Used by permission of Tyndale House Publishers. All rights reserved. (referred to in this book as NLT)

Idahosa, Chizabam, Understanding the Role of the Holy Spirit as our Helper, https://beautifulinjesus.com/holy-spirit-helper/, "Tues 14th" is only date provided.

Lucado, Max, *You'll Get Through This*, Thomas Nelson; Copyright

Merriam-Webster Dictionary. https://www.merriam-webster.com/dictionary all words were found on this site.

Nelson, Matt, *The Beauty of the In-Between,* Self-Published by City Church, Tulsa, OK. ISBN 978-1-7337667-0-8. Copyright 2019

PC Study Bible 4 Software. No other information found.

Peterson, Eugene H., *THE MESSAGE: The Bible in Contemporary Language*; Copyright 2002 (referred to in this book as MSG)

Smedes, Lewis B. *Forgive and Forget: Healing the Hurts We Don't Deserve;* ISBN 978-0-06-128582-0 New York, NY
HarperCollins Publishers; www.harpercollins.com
Copyright 1984, 1996.

Subotnik, Rona B., and Gloria Harris. *Surviving Infidelity; Making Decisions, Recovering from the Pain.* Adams Media, 2005

Urban Dictionary. *Godwink*. Last updated by Kimber E October 7, 2007,
https://www.urbandictionary.com/define.php?term=godwink

Walton, Owen, *The Holy Spirit our Helper; Parakletos,*
https://exceedingfaith.com/holy-spirit-helper-parakletos/
updated on March 29, 2019

Wikipedia.org, *Butterfly Effect; Web.*
https://en.wikipedia.org/wiki/Butterfly_effect; last updated July 18, 2020. Retrieved July 26, 2020

Wiktionary.org, *God wink; Web.*
https://en.wiktionary.org/wiki/God_wink; last updated September 28, 2019. Retrieved October 16, 2020.

*I have tried to give credit where credit is due, however, there are times I take notes and forget to write down who said what and the date. If I have failed to list a name or citation, please forgive me. I truly made an effort to cite accurately, but there were times I could not find or remember where I heard it.

Author's Bio

Sandy Sue Spaan Sheaffer was born and raised in Oklahoma City, Oklahoma. She graduated from Putnam City High School and attended OU. She married her high school sweetheart and worked with him 30+ years. After their divorce she went back to school and earned an Associates in Business from OCCC and a certificate of ministry in the Assemblies of God in 2009. She attained her Bachelor of Business Administration in 2012 but continued until she achieved her MBA in 2014. That same year she received her teaching certificate, fulfilling a lifelong dream to teach. She currently teaches 7th grade Reading and Advanced Literature at Newcastle Middle School in the Newcastle Public School District. She previously taught English at Brink Junior High in the Moore Public Schools District.

Sandy is the mother of three children: 2 sons, Doc and Duke, and a daughter, Sesily. She considers Doc's wife, Cami, and Sesily's husband, Josh, hers also. She is the grandmother of Doc and Cami's two children, Trip and Shaylee, and Josh and Sesily's two boys, Shane and Shepherd.

Sandy spent many years as a self-proclaimed "professional volunteer" serving her church and the local PTA's where her children attended school. She was also on the Board of Directors for the Southwest Integris Medical Center Foundation, the SW Integris

Scoliosis Foundation, and served as Secretary on the Moore Public School Foundation for 13+ years.

For over 30 years Sandy was active in her church's music program as both a musician and a singer. She also worked in the church office, coordinated weddings, and produced the weekly bulletin. Sandy has been on numerous mission trips around the world, 19 to Africa alone, participating in church planting crusades. Most of all she loves to spend time with her family and friends.

Ms. Sheaffer has also authored and published two other books:

Babies Should Come w/ Instructions
Mail $10 per book (includes shipping and handling) payable to:
Dewey Productions
2701 SW 139th Street
Oklahoma City, OK 73170

Adolescents: Over 100+ stories to make parents feel better about their teens and young adults (available for download on Amazon)

Made in the USA
Coppell, TX
05 September 2023

21236045R00115